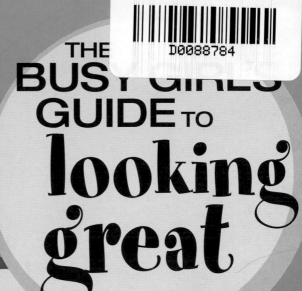

THE BUSY GIRLS GUIDE TO looking great

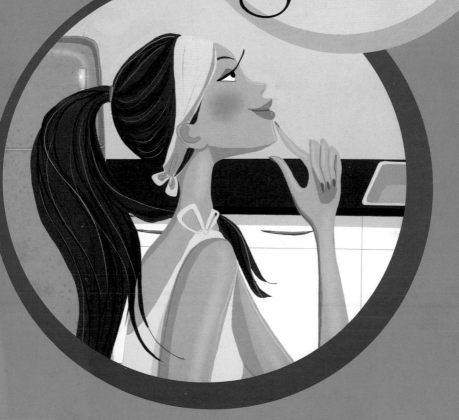

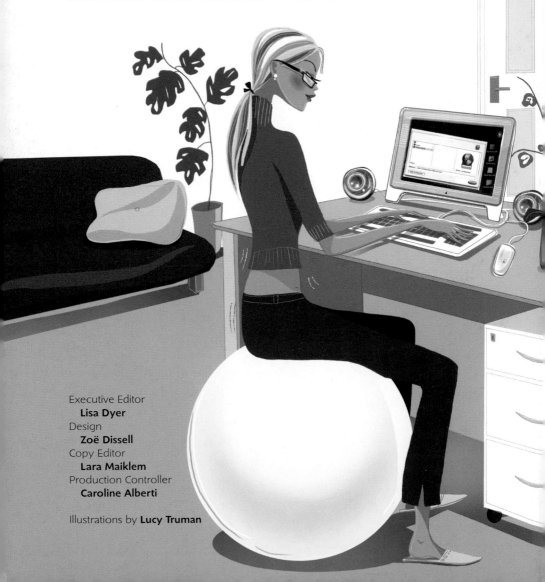

Executive Editor
Lisa Dyer
Design
Zoë Dissell
Copy Editor
Lara Maiklem
Production Controller
Caroline Alberti

Illustrations by **Lucy Truman**

THE BUSY GIRL'S GUIDE TO looking great

CAROLINE JONES

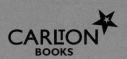

CARLTON
BOOKS

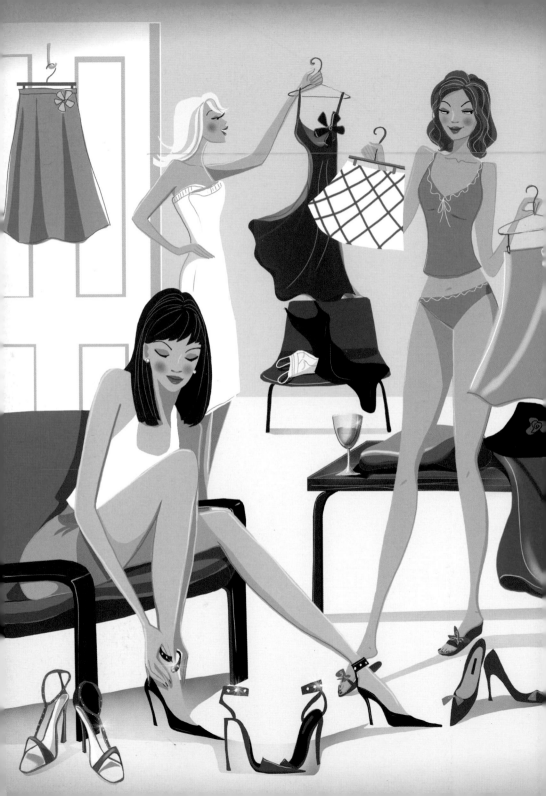

CONTENTS

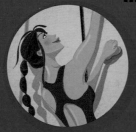
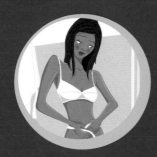
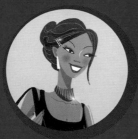
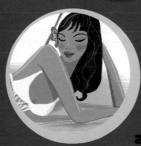

INTRODUCTION

Calling on busy girls everywhere – here at last is a
guide dedicated to making sure you can have it all.

Sadly, when the going gets tough, most women don't go
shopping. Instead we sacrifice all those little luxuries that
make us feel beautiful, such as facials, yoga classes, shoe
shopping and healthy cooking. And the end result? We
feel frazzled, unpolished and downright unhealthy.

It's all very well being a celebrity with your own
nutritionist, personal trainer, make-up artist and stylist,
plus the time to work on looking fabulous. But how's
a real girl supposed to compete when she has work, a
hectic social life, and relationship and family demands to
juggle? Well, the good news is, you need struggle no
longer. This book has been written to help you achieve
all your health and beauty desires – without derailing
your frantic schedule.

HAVE YOU **EVER** DONE ANY OF **THE FOLLOWING?**

✿ Tried to apply make-up on the journey to work?
✿ Skipped the gym because you had to work late?
✿ Eaten takeout three nights in a row because you were too tired to cook?
✿ Worn an unflattering, out-of-date dress because it's the only thing clean?

IF SO, THEN THIS IS **THE BOOK** FOR YOU.

Whether you're a single girl or a working mother, this fun,
information-filled guide will show you how to incorporate
exercise into your day, stick to a healthy diet and look
stylish and groomed – all effortlessly and in the minimum
amount of time.

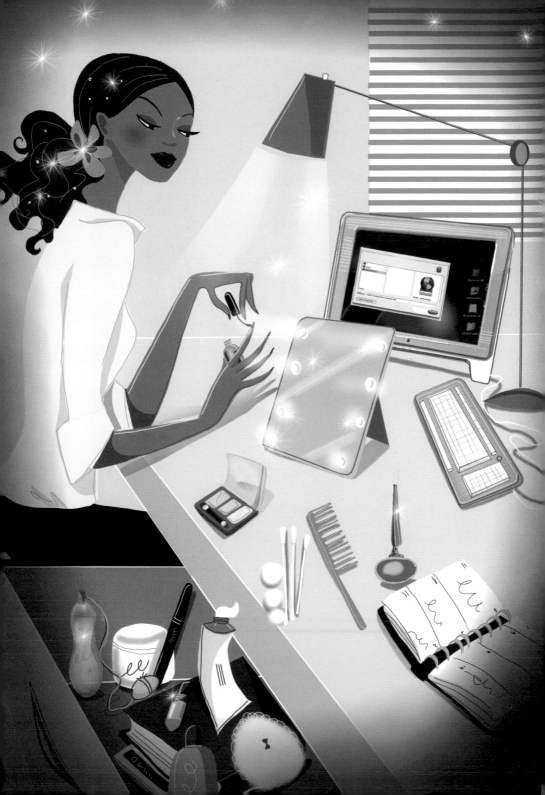

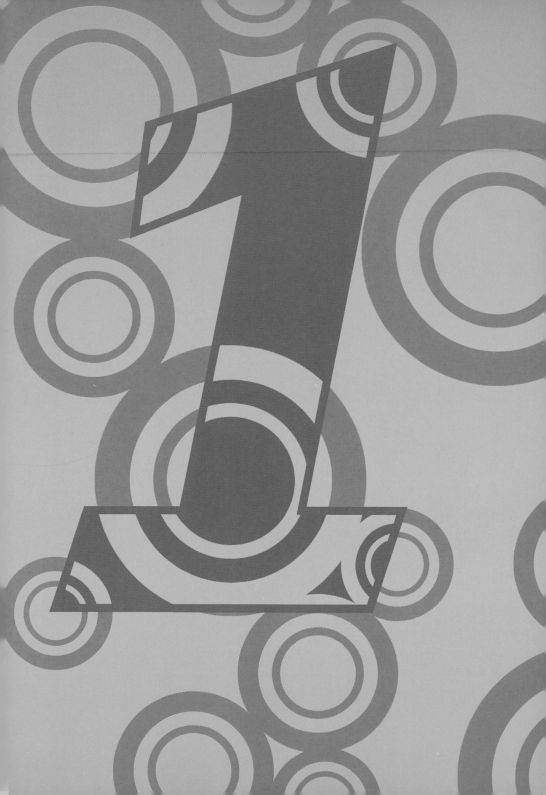

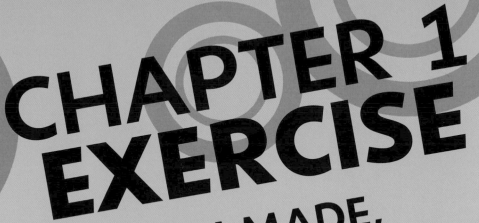

CHAPTER 1
EXERCISE
DECISION MADE, TIME FOR ACTION

Here's how to get **motivated** and get **moving**. Your foolproof plan to achieve the **body** you've always **dreamed** of – without spending hours at the **gym**.

Exercise is the **easiest** way to improve your health and body shape: it will help you live longer, boost your self-esteem and make you feel generally **happier** and full of **energy**. But while you know how important exercise is and you really do want to **get fit**, your schedule already seems to be bursting at the seams, and you don't think you could fit in even one more **activity!** Does this sound familiar? Take heart – the hardest part about taking regular exercise is getting started and the first few weeks are always the most difficult. Not only are you not in **shape**, you're also trying to adjust to a new routine.

Unfortunately, many of those who start an **exercise programme** give up within a few weeks and never achieve their goals. Here you'll find the **tips** you need to stick with it and see quick results. Studies have been done which prove that if you make it past the first two months, you're likely to continue to **exercise** long term. What's more, once you get into working out regularly, the chances are that you'll discover you **love it** and can't do without it. And no matter how busy your lifestyle, it's always easier to find time for something you enjoy.

First, **decide** what you want out of exercise and set yourself some realistic **goals**. Having a specific fitness plan will make exercise easier to organize. Remember to check with your doctor before starting on any **fitness** regime, particularly if you are pregnant or have any existing health conditions or injuries.

HOW TO **GET STARTED**

Use that inner voice telling you to get moving to work up a programme for action.

PLAN IT ON PAPER

Once you've identified your specific fitness goals, draw up a plan of attack. Laying out your objectives like this will give you a **visual reminder** to help you to stay focused, organized and in control. Putting it in writing will also make your plan feel more formal and will encourage you to take it seriously.

SET YOURSELF **REALISTIC** GOALS

Even one session a week is a success, because it means that you're actually committing to **regular exercise**. You can build on the frequency of the visits from there. Not everyone can fit in the 'desirable' three times a week so don't beat yourself up if you can't manage it. Just tell yourself that twice a week is good and three times is simply fantastic.

★**TIP** Pick a special event about two months away and plan the outfit you want to wear and the size you hope to buy it in. Visualizing how great you'll look will give you a strong incentive to stick to your exercise regime.

SET A DAY OF **RECKONING**

Write down the exact date you want to **achieve** your goals. If you don't, it leaves you wide open to some non-specified time in the future, which you'll keep pushing back and probably never reach.

TELL SOMEONE ELSE

If you confide in a friend or partner about your plans, you'll be more likely to achieve **success** – you'll feel compelled to stick to it because you won't want to lose face by giving up!

PENCIL **YOURSELF** IN

Undoubtedly you will have busy days when you won't be able to exercise **spontaneously**, so you need to plan ahead. Be firm and schedule exercise into your diary as if it's an important meeting that can't be missed.

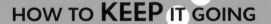

HOW TO **KEEP** IT GOING

Finding a way, every day, to make it easy to exercise will keep you **motivated** and focused long-term.

BREAK IT UP

You don't have to do your whole workout in one go. If you're too busy to take a whole hour out of your day, you can get exactly the same benefits by exercising sporadically throughout the day. Try **15 minutes** when you wake up, 15 minutes at lunchtime and 15 minutes last thing at night. Before you know it, you'll have clocked up 45 minutes of exercise that day.

EASY DOES IT

Get into an exercise routine gradually or you could injure yourself – and the chances are that you'll burn yourself out too quickly. If you're not a regular gym-goer, begin with something easy, such as brisk walking – even a **short walk** will give your heart, lungs and leg muscles a good workout. Start by walking for 5–10 minutes a day and build this up, bit by bit, adding 2–3 minutes each time.

DON'T EXPECT INSTANT **RESULTS**

Exercise won't change your body overnight, so even if you can't **see a difference** after the first week or two, don't get disappointed and give up. It generally takes a month before your body shape starts to change and something between three and six months to achieve optimum results.

You will notice other benefits, too. Along with increased energy levels, you will start feeling less stressed and generally **happier**, so be sure to register the improvements when you notice them. Keeping the benefits in mind will keep you motivated.

Motivation **checklist**

★ Find a form of exercise that is both enjoyable and convenient. So, if you hate running, don't start a running programme: try brisk walking instead. Similarly, even if you enjoy swimming, it's not a good choice if you don't have easy access to a pool.

★ If you change into your workout clothes even when you don't feel like exercising, the chances are that you'll go ahead and break into a sweat – seeing as how you're all ready and dressed for it!

★ Visualize how good you're going to feel when you've finished your workout, and then go and make it happen. Believe that it will be the best thing you do all day.

★ Choose your most positive friend as your 'motivator'. Tell them your fitness goals and ask them to encourage you when you're flagging. A quick reminder of what you're trying to achieve by a third party can work wonders!

★ Change the order of your workout or the main emphasis to keep interest.

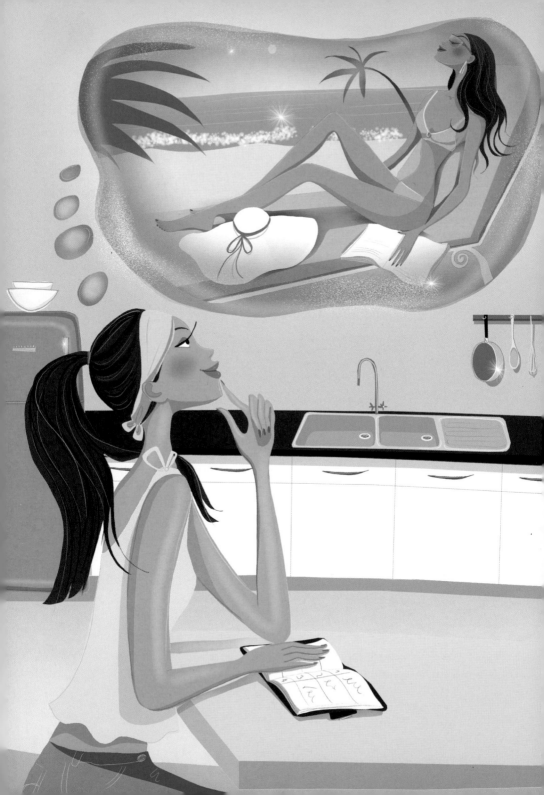

REWARD YOURSELF

There's nothing like a reward to make you feel good about what you've achieved and to help to keep you motivated. Give **yourself a treat** for every step of your fitness plan that you achieve. Try to choose things that aren't food-based – that new top you've had your eye on or a book you've wanted to read for ages, perhaps. Then plan a really special reward for when you've reached your ultimate target – maybe an **exotic trip** or a pair of Manolo Blahnik heels.

How much exercise is enough?

Reports from the *Journal of the American Medical Association* and studies at Duke University, North Carolina, show that 30 minutes of moderate exercise every day is enough to keep you in shape. But don't panic, this doesn't mean you have to spend every day at the gym. Walking, stair climbing, cleaning – and any other daily activities that require a bit of effort – all count towards this total. Even so, a staggering seven out of ten women (70 per cent) don't take enough exercise to benefit their health or to keep themselves slim.

Top ten benefits of being fit

1 More confidence about your body and body image.
2 Healthier heart and lungs.
3 Stronger bones and joints, which will reduce the risk of developing osteoporosis, the bone-thinning disease.
4 Stress levels will be slashed.
5 Sleep quality will improve.
6 You'll feel happier and be less likely to suffer depression.
7 Energy levels will increase.
8 Your brain will be sharper and faster-working.
9 You'll be less at risk of developing most cancers – including breast cancer.
10 You'll be less likely to suffer with back problems as you get older.

FITNESS MYTHS
UNCOVERED

There are lots of myths about getting fit, which can be enough to put you off before you've even started. Thankfully, most of them simply aren't true. For example, many people think you have to be in real pain to get any benefit from exercise or that you need to dedicate all your free time if you want to get in shape. Neither are correct, and here are some more myths to watch out for.

MYTH 1: IF YOU WORKOUT, YOU CAN EAT AS MUCH AS YOU LIKE

False. You can't fill up on high-fat, sugary foods just because you're exercising. If you want to lose weight and keep it off, you need to combine a healthy **balanced diet** with exercise, which means eating less fat, less sugar and more fruits and vegetables.

MYTH 2: TO GET FIT YOU NEED TO GO TO THE GYM EVERY DAY

False. As little as 30 minutes a day is enough to keep you in tip-top shape.

MYTH 3: WOMEN WHO **LIFT WEIGHTS** GET HUGE MUSCLES

False. Women simply don't have enough testosterone to develop large, **bulky muscles**. Strength training with light weights doesn't cause women to build muscles – only taking steroids can do that.

MYTH 4: SPOT **REDUCING** IS POSSIBLE

False. Sadly, you can't 'burn off' fat in one specific area of your body by exercising that particular part. Even if **toning exercises** will tighten muscles and give you more definition, only the combination of regular aerobic exercise and a low-fat diet can actually shift body fat.

MYTH 5: NO **PAIN**, NO **GAIN**

False. Exercising to the point of pain does not help you and can actually cause you serious physical harm. It's important to **push yourself** a bit, in order to strengthen your heart, lungs and muscles, but if you're not careful, you could injure yourself. Exercise should never cause physical pain.

MYTH 6: MUSCLE WEIGHS **MORE THAN FAT**, SO THE FITTER YOU ARE, THE HEAVIER YOU ARE

False. Muscle doesn't actually weigh more than body fat; it is **denser**, though, so one pound of muscle will take up much less room in your body than one pound of fat. What's more, muscle provides a better blood supply than body fat and so burns more calories – even while at rest.

WHAT'S YOUR FITNESS PERSONALITY?

If you're like most people, you'll probably have joined a gym at least once in your life but, for whatever reason, you don't go any more. Maybe you got bored or perhaps you just couldn't find the time to go. One of the problems about exercise is that the generally held belief that 'one size fits all' doesn't take into account how busy your job is or what kind of person you are, and consequently you can waste time and energy trying to make the wrong kind of workout work for you. In order to find your perfect exercise regime – which you will enjoy and stick to – you need to delve a bit deeper into what makes you tick.

This quiz will help you to discover the best type of workout plan to keep you motivated and get you in shape.

Q1 WHAT'S THE MAIN REASON YOU WANT TO EXERCISE?

A To maintain a high level of fitness.

B To burn calories and lose weight.

C To relax and escape from stress.

D To meet new people.

Q2 WHAT'S YOUR IDEA OF A PERFECT HOLIDAY?

A An active break with plenty of water sports or sailing.

B A quiet cruise that involves lots of lazing around by the pool.

C Somewhere that exercise can be combined with exploring the local culture.

D A resort with a busy nightlife.

Q3 WHAT DO YOU MOST FEEL LIKE DOING AFTER A STRESSFUL WEEK AT WORK?

A Having a cleaning blitz to work all the tension out of your system.

B Having a long lie-in on Saturday.

C Having a long walk in the country.

D Having a big night out with friends.

Q4 WHAT DO YOU CONSIDER A GOOD WORKOUT?

A One that leaves me aching and sweating.

B Just making it to the gym is an achievement for me!

C One that leaves me calm and relaxed.

D One when I meet lots of new people.

Q5 WHAT'S YOUR DIET LIKE?

A I buy lots of low-calorie, low-fat foods.

B I'm very busy so I eat a lot of microwave meals.

C Very healthy – lots of fruit, vegetables and whole grains.

D I eat normally during the day, but often skip dinner if I'm going out.

Q6 WHICH STATEMENT BEST DESCRIBES YOU?

A Ambitious, but fair-minded.

B Hard-working and often stressed.

C Caring and laidback.

D Extrovert and fun loving.

MOSTLY 'A'S – THE **EXERCISE-AHOLIC**

The rest of your life fits in around your visits to the gym or training sessions for your latest fitness-based event – whether it's a race or a sponsored swim. You enjoy running, spinning and circuit training – basically anything that means you can push your body to the limit. You're always looking for a new fitness craze to try and feel restless and irritable if you **miss a gym session**. Exercise is something you prefer to do alone and you take it very seriously.

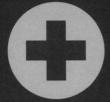

Potential **problems**

Continue like this and you'll suffer from burnout and risk an injury. Plus, **boredom** may set in and you'll find that you'll begin to get less out of gym visits.

Making it **work** for you

Lighten up! Put the fun back into your gym sessions by trying something a bit **less intense**, but just as challenging, such as salsa or belly-dancing lessons. Spending time doing classes, instead of just putting in solitary gym sessions, will open up the social side of exercise to you. It would also benefit you to mix your high-energy workouts with something more gentle and relaxing to help you unwind. Your body needs time to rest and recover after **intensive** exercise, so try to incorporate some stretching or Pilates classes into your weekly programme. This will help lengthen your muscles, improve your flexibility and reduce your stress levels.

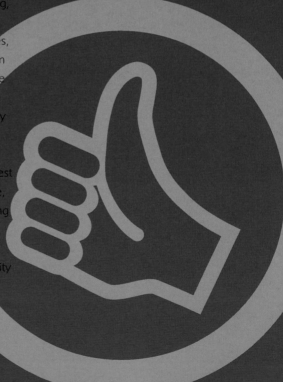

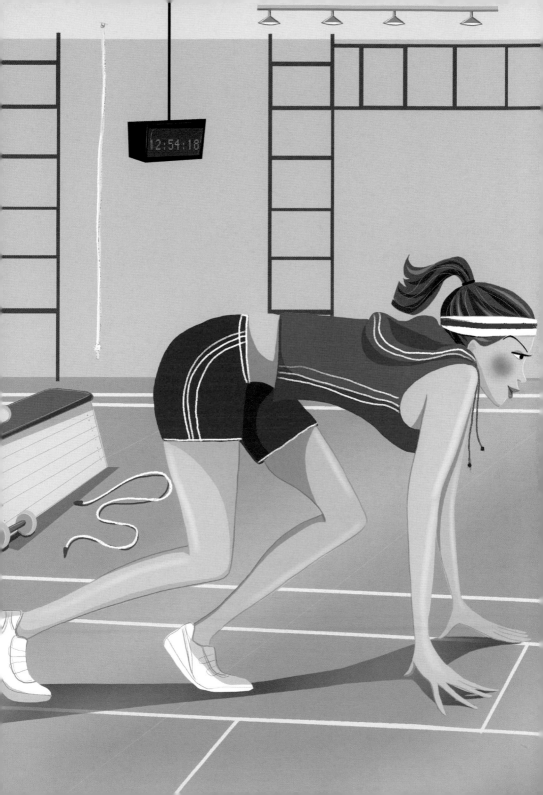

MOSTLY 'B'S – **THE STRESS BUNNY**

Joining the gym seemed like a great idea at the time, but the demands of a hectic lifestyle – including **work, family and friends** – means that you find it almost impossible to establish a regular fitness routine. Your intentions are great, but if you do manage to **get to the gym** or find time to put on a fitness video, it's a miracle.

Potential **problems**

You're always likely to put off getting fit to some date in the future that never actually arrives. The truth is, if you join a gym and don't start going regularly because you're **too busy**, or buy a fitness video and don't play it in the first week, the chances are high that you never will. So you will have wasted your money and won't get fit.

Making it work for **you**

You have to learn to make exercise a priority. Ultra-busy people often see going to the gym – or even working out at home – as an indulgence that they shouldn't waste time on. But this is simply not the case. Being fit will keep you healthy, help you look and feel better, and make you perform more efficiently in all the other areas of your life. Look upon exercise as a necessity. If you're really time-poor, a **personal trainer** may help you to focus on your goals and organize your day better, while classes such as yoga and t'ai chi will also **reduce your stress** levels.

★**TIP** Log onto Ebay and scan for a second-hand cross-training machine that you can jump on for 10 minutes each morning before you shower. They're better than exercise bikes as they work the entire body.

MOSTLY C'S – THE ZEN GODDESS

Exercise, for you, is just one part of your holistic lifestyle. You love eating healthily, so try to stick to natural, organic foods and enjoy getting in touch with your **spiritual side**. In fact, toning up your inner peace is more important to you than firming up your inner thighs. This means that, while you love long walks in the country and practise yoga regularly, you never work up a real sweat with any aerobic exercise.

Potential problems

While yoga has plenty of great health benefits and will give you a toned, flexible body, it won't provide your heart and lungs with a workout. So if this is the only form of exercise you take, your actual fitness levels will be quite low and you won't benefit from the reduced risk of heart disease and other serious illness that go hand in hand with **cardiovascular exercise**. Although brisk walks will help to boost your level of cardiovascular fitness, they need to be a regular feature of your week to make any difference. And bear in mind that, if you want to lose weight, yoga and Pilates are not fat-burning forms of exercise so although they will tone the body shape, they will not actually shift excess weight.

How to keep motivated

Alternating yoga with higher-impact cardio classes will improve your stamina and flexibility, which will in turn boost your yoga potential. If you are looking to shift excess pounds, you'll need to **raise the tempo** of your workout. Try something like kickboxing or jazz dancing, which should appeal to your creative side. Cycling or jogging at weekends are also ideal, as they allow you to indulge your love of the countryside, giving your heart a good workout at the same time.

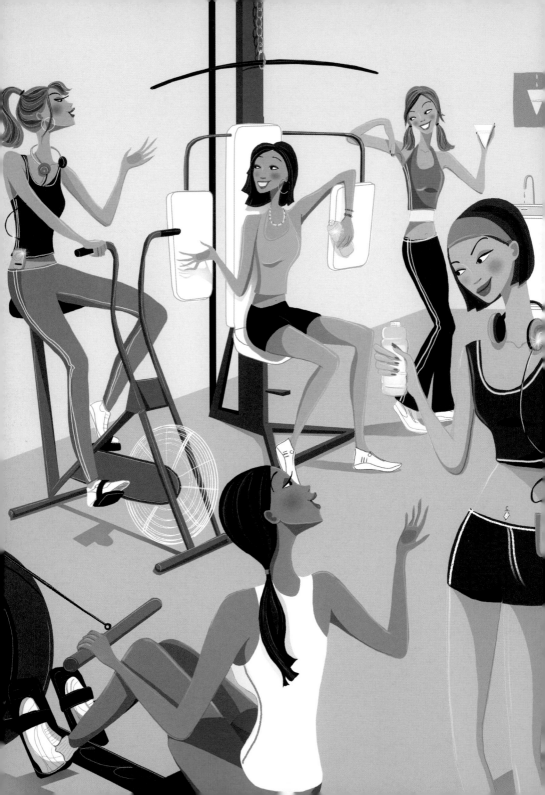

MOSTLY 'D'S – **THE SOCIAL BUTTERFLY**

For you, the best bit about going to the gym or joining a sports club is the chance to socialize and meet new people. On the downside, this can mean that despite the fact that you go regularly, real exercise is pretty low on your agenda because you spend most of your time chatting and having a laugh.

Potential **problems**

While getting fit should be fun, exercising your jaw more than the rest of your body means that you're not actually improving your fitness levels or getting your body in shape! A good exercise programme should combine sessions where you work alone – lifting weights or doing stretches, for example – with **team sports** or classes shared with other people. Too much emphasis on one or the other can lead to an unbalanced regime and may result in boredom and/or poor results.

How to **keep** motivated

Find out if your workplace organizes team sports, such as netball or hockey, which enjoy a good social scene and where you'll meet new people – the social life of the sport usually extends way beyond the court. Alternatively, find a gym that offers these activities. As an **extrovert**, you'll also benefit from attending fun but challenging classes available at your gym, because the group atmosphere will encourage you to work harder.

Arrange to meet friends from your gym for drinks after a workout. This will give you something to look forward to so that you'll waste less time chatting when you should be exercising!

How to make exercise work for you

1 Find a gym close to home or the office. If it's any more than 10 minutes away it'll be too easy to find excuses not to go.

2 Get a friend to join with you. Not only will it be more fun, but you'll be able to give each other encouragement and you'll also feel guilty about letting them down if you don't go.

3 Think about when you feel most active. Be honest with yourself. If you're not a morning person, then there's no point in planning a programme that means you have to exercise before work as you won't stick to it. Likewise, if you're a morning person, fit a session into the first half of your day – don't force yourself to exercise after work.

4 'I'm too tired' is no good as an excuse. Exercise gives you more energy, which means in the long run you'll feel less drained. Plus it releases 'feel-good' endorphins into the brain so you'll feel happier and less stressed after a workout.

5 Reward yourself after a gym session with a sauna or a little treat, such as a new body lotion or a magazine.

FIT IN FITNESS,
WHATEVER YOUR LIFESTYLE

YOU WORK PART-TIME

If your working hours are fairly **flexible**, you should find it easy to combine regular workouts with the odd spontaneous session.

Try

- Joining a gym. Your lifestyle means you can use it a lot, which makes it worth the money. If you use the gym outside its busiest times, it's worth looking for one that offers discounted 'off-peak' membership.
- If you find you have an hour to fill unexpectedly, use it wisely and go for a run or swim.
- If you work afternoons, make the most of early-morning sessions at the gym or pool. Exercising in the morning will also boost your metabolism for the rest of the day.

YOU'RE A BUSY MOTHER

If you're rushing around a lot, without much structure to your day, it can be hard to fit in exercise. Anyway, you're probably exhausted by trying to **juggle everything** already, so just the thought of working out seems a chore – and a full-time job quite appealing at times!

Try

- Incorporating exercise into your daily routine. Run up and down the stairs, fit in a few sit-ups while the children's supper is cooking, or jog on the spot.
- Join a class, like yoga, that you can still practise on your own at home if you have to miss a session because you're too busy.
- If you work as well, try to fit a swim or 45-minute run into your lunch hour to utilize the time when you're not looking after the kids.

YOU WORK **REGULAR** HOURS

If your working hours are predictable, it should be easy
for you to fit exercise into your routine. The predictability,
however, may lead to a lack of **motivation**, making it hard
for you to stick to a regime for long.

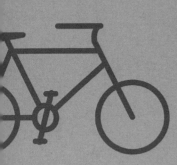

Try
- Walking or cycling to work every other day – you'll
  boost your fitness levels and save money.
- Pre-paying to join a course of lunchtime or post-work
  yoga classes. If it's already paid for, you'll be less likely
  to skip a class unless you have a really good reason.
- Making exercise a social event and organize going
  for a bike ride with friends at the weekend.

YOU WORK LONG, **IRREGULAR** HOURS

You start work early and often finish after the gym has closed. Sometimes
you have to work weekends as well, which means that exercise goes entirely
out of the window. Trying to fit regular workouts into your **hectic life** can be a
scheduling nightmare.

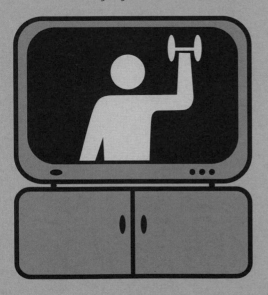

Try
- Fitting in as much brisk walking as
  possible. Lots of small segments
  of cumulative exercise are just as
  good as long sessions – they all
  add up.
- Invest in a fitness video or book
  and make a pact with yourself
  to work with that at least once
  a week. Then you can consider
  any additional exercise a bonus.
- If you sit hunched in front of a
  computer all day, don't forget to
  get up and stretch every hour or
  so to prevent postural problems.

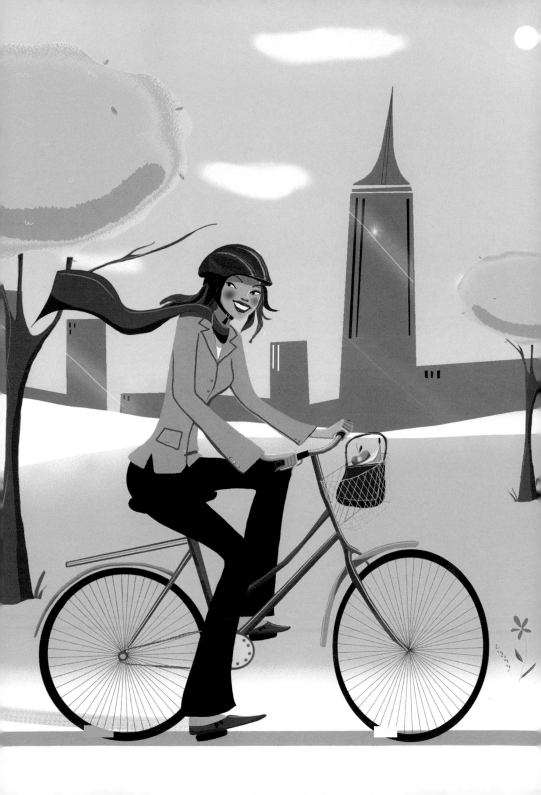

LUNCH-BREAK FITNESS

Whether you have a busy social life, young kids, a long working day or a combination of all three, your lunch hour is often the most convenient time to exercise. But getting there, changing, working out, showering and getting back to the office all has to happen in that hour, too. That time has to work hard for you. How do you make it really count?

If you do want to workout in your lunch hour, it's a good idea to think of activities involving **minimal sweat** so that you don't have to waste precious time in the changing rooms. In fact, with a little forward planning, there are lots of clever ways you can fit exercise into that hour.

SWIMMING

Good idea

Swimming's a great idea if you're a bit of a water baby who loves thrashing out a few lengths in the pool, and is ideal if you have knee, ankle or shoulder injuries, because the resistance of the water means there is **no pressure** on your joints.

Bad idea

Don't swim if you take ages to get ready and **dry your hair**. Not only will you spend half your time in the changing room, but you will also feel rushed and harassed by the time you get back to the office.

POWER WALKING

Good idea

Walking uphill on the treadmill is great for **toning** calves, thighs and bottom muscles and you won't get as sweaty as you do when you run.

Bad idea

It's not so good if fitness equipment, such as the treadmill, tends to bore you, because you'll be less likely to make the commitment to go.

LIFTING WEIGHTS

Good idea

Lifting a few light weights at lunchtime will not only increase your lean muscle mass and boost your metabolism, which will help you **burn more fat** and calories, but also help you end up with lean, sculpted arms and legs – without too much of a sweat, either.

Bad idea

If you have any existing injuries or if you lifted weights yesterday, your muscles need a day to recover.

YOGA AND PILATES
Good idea
Both these activities will improve your strength, flexibility and muscle tone. What's more, they can do it without getting you all hot and bothered, so you won't need to shower afterwards. Plus, they will **slash your stress levels** if you're having a bad day.

Bad idea
If you're exercising as part of a weight-loss programme, you'd be better off trading in a 45-minute yoga class for 30 minutes' cardio work, using the saved 15 minutes to shower and get ready for whatever you're doing next.

GOING FOR A WALK
Good idea
If the weather's good and you're wearing suitable shoes (not kitten heels, that is!), **walking briskly** will burn a fair number of calories. You'll also give yourself a boosting dose of vitamin D, the nutrient that's produced when **sunlight** hits your skin – and low levels of vitamin D have been linked to depression.

Bad idea
If it's raining or really cold outside, you'll soon find an excuse not to go or, if you do set off, you then won't spend long enough walking to get any real benefit.

★**TIP** **If you have to work through lunch, take a 20-minute coffee break later in the afternoon when things have quietened down – but skip the caffeine fix and go for a brisk walk instead.**

Five ways to make lunchtime exercise a cinch

1 Arrange with your boss to take an early lunch at midday or a late one at 2 pm, so that you can avoid the gym's peak busy time between 12 pm and 2 pm.

2 Choose a gym as near as possible to work, so that your time is spent exercising, not in getting there and back.

3 Take advantage of the complimentary clean towels provided by many gyms to save the hassle of taking your own.

4 Think you're too busy to leave your desk? Remember, exercise helps to reduce stress levels and boosts energy. Research has found that employees are more productive in the afternoon if they workout in their lunch hour.

5 Remind yourself that by exercising at lunch, rather than putting it off until after work, you'll feel great at 5.30 pm when you can go straight home – or out on the town!

DOUBLE-DUTY EXERCISE

Do you have a gym membership you never use? Have you bought home fitness equipment that's gathering dust in the corner? Have you broken **every resolution** to get fit you've ever made because you can't seem to find the time? Don't worry. You can still achieve those fitness goals – all it takes is a little rescheduling and some clever planning. Start by keeping a diary of how you spend your free time and then **sit down and analyse** it at the end of the week. You may find that you can slot an extra 30 minutes into your day or you can be wiser about how much time you spend on daily tasks and chores. Do you really need to watch so much TV in the evening, for example, or perhaps you could wash and dry your hair at night to free up some time in the morning?

One of the best ways to introduce more exercise into your life is to treat your chosen activity as a multitasking opportunity. There are various ways in which you can get exercise to perform a double duty in your life.

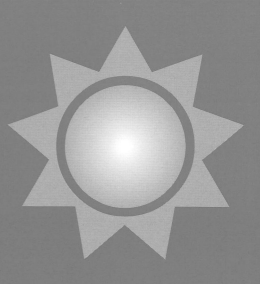

SWIM FOR **CHARITY**

If a lot of your time seems to be taken up by commitments to various organizations and helping others, and you're the sort of person who can't say 'no' to any sort of volunteer work, then try to find ways to make that work for you fitness-wise as well. **Sponsored swims**, triathlons and walks all require months of training beforehand – and they are always for a good cause. What better way (or reason) to keep fit?

BE A **TEAM** PLAYER

Joining the company sports team – be it football or softball – provides a great combination of networking, fun and exercise. It can make you seem more approachable to colleagues and boost your confidence, while improving **teamwork skills** at the same time.

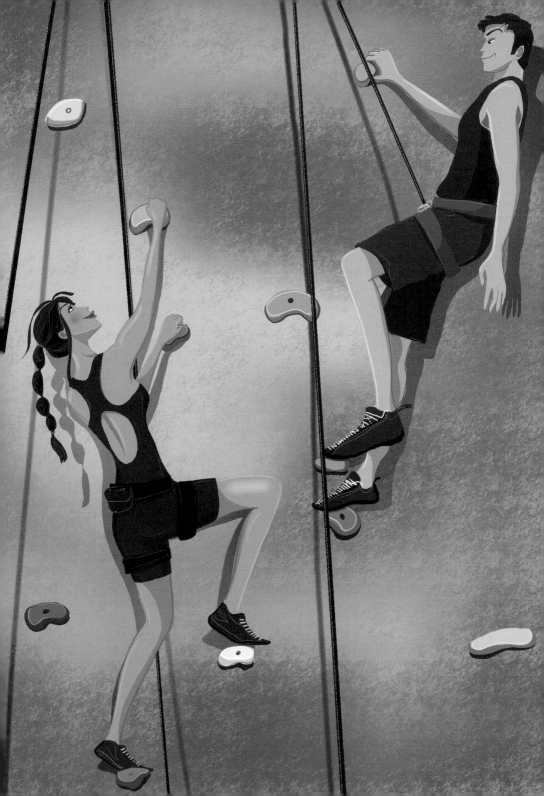

RUN AN **ERRAND**

Rushing around for your entire lunch hour endeavouring to pay bills, do a little food shopping, pick up a birthday card and drop off some dry-cleaning will burn plenty of calories. And – big bonus! – it helps to get the rest of your life under control so that you can relax and unwind in the evening or be free to **go out and socialize**.

★**TIP** **Using lunchtime to do a supermarket sweep? Up the effort factor by choosing to shop somewhere that's a good 10-minute walk from the office.**

DATE-A-**MATE**

Whether you're just friends, in a more solid relationship, or on the lookout, sports activities that combine the social with the physical are a great way to bond. Joining a running, rock-climbing or tennis club will also help you to meet new people with similar interests – potential friends and motivators. Suggesting a tennis match or an afternoon's ice-skating as a first date is a great, fun way to take the awkwardness out of the situation. Plus, the energy rush has an **aphrodisiac effect** and you'll soon discover what he's really like by the way he plays the game!

LEND **A HAND**

Do you have a friend who's about to move, or one who needs some help painting her living room? Is someone in your family yearning to sort out their mess of a garden, but not able to face tackling it alone? If so, volunteer to help – carrying boxes and furniture can be like a session in the weight room. Make sure you do some **light stretching** before and afterwards, and be careful not to strain your back. Not only will you **burn fat** and work all your large muscle groups, you'll also score points with your friends and family, and probably get a buzz from knowing you've helped someone out, too.

GET SOME FOUR-LEGGED **ENCOURAGEMENT**

If you're looking for an incentive to exercise, you could rescue an abandoned dog from an animal centre. You'll feel good about providing a much-needed home and, because dogs have to be walked every day, you'll have **no excuse** but to get fit.

Start with a regular 30-minute walk. Then, once your dog gets in the habit of walking with you, he will beg to spend that time with you – and you'll find it impossible to say no if you look into those **big brown eyes**. Plus, there must be further hidden health benefits too, because studies show that people who own pets live longer than those who don't: pet owning leads to a reduction in **stress levels** and lower blood pressure.

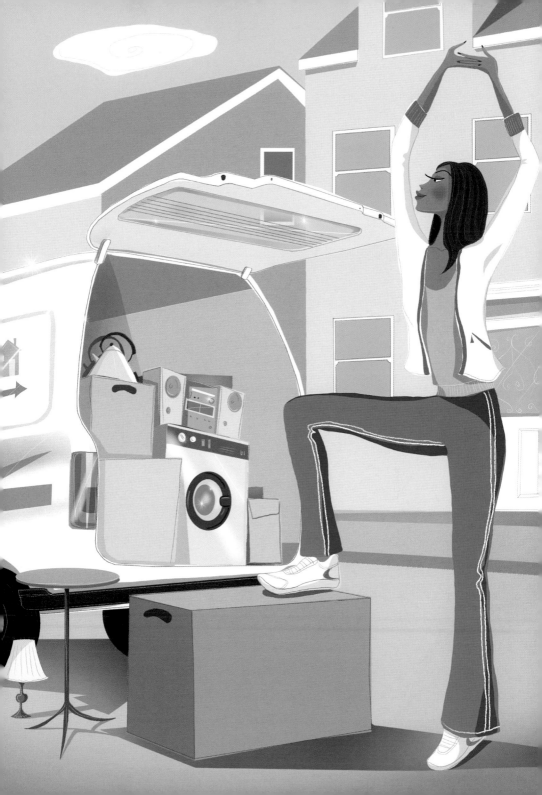

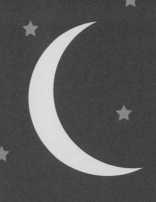

LOOK MORE TONED BY
TONIGHT

It's seven o'clock, you're going out in an hour and you want to look your best but you're feeling a bit flabby and it's too late to diet now. Don't panic! There is an alternative. As an emergency quick fix, try this easy workout; it will temporarily pump up and tighten all your muscles, so that you look more toned than you really are when your hot date arrives. And the great thing is, you don't have to get to the gym – all the moves can be done at home.

WHAT IT DOES AND HOW IT DOES IT

These five key exercises will 'spot tone' your body – fast. They provide your muscles with pump and definition, giving your body a firmer, more streamlined look in your party outfit.

This method works on the **'pump principle'** by forcing blood into your muscles and pumping them up, thus improving their definition and making them look tighter and feel more toned in the short term. Although doing these moves an hour before you go out will help you look great for a couple of hours that night, doing them more regularly will produce longer-lasting results.

YOUR **15-MINUTE** WORKOUT

Forget fiddly workout routines and fancy gym equipment, you can do these simple moves anywhere – even while you're watching TV!

For **SCULPTED** calves

Stand with your feet just over hip-width apart and turned out slightly. Cross your arms in front of your chest. Look ahead and **breathe in** as you bend your knees to make a right angle, lowering your body but keeping your back upright and straight. Then straighten your legs as you exhale. Repeat 25 times.

For **TIGHTER** buttocks

Lie on your back, with your knees bent and slightly apart. Your feet should be flat on the floor, arms at your sides and your hips raised slightly off the floor. Keep your **abs pulled in**. Breathe out as you raise your hips slightly higher and squeeze your bottom muscles together hard. Inhale and lower your back down to your starting position. Repeat 25 times.

For better-toned **ARMS**

Find a safe, solid chair and place your hands over the edge, roughly hip-width apart. Then move slightly away from the chair so that your body weight is evenly distributed between your arms and feet. Keep your hips low and your knees bent and look ahead. Inhale and bend your elbows so that they're at **right angles**, keeping them slightly tucked in. To complete the exercise, half-straighten your arms as you breathe out. Repeat 25 times.

For flatter **ABS**

Lie on your back with both legs lifted up from the hips until they are at right angles to the floor, toes pointing to the ceiling. **Support your head** with a hand by each ear. Raise your head and shoulders off the floor and keep them lifted throughout the exercise. Twist your upper body so that your right elbow meets your left knee. Return to the centre. Then twist to the other side, your left elbow rising to meet your right knee. Repeat 25 times on each side.

For **SLIMMER** thighs

Lie on the floor with your hands under your buttocks for support, keeping your head back, your feet flexed and your knees slightly bent. Slowly open your legs out to the sides as far as is comfortable, breathing out as you do so. Then to return, gradually bring your legs together as you inhale. Make sure you keep your **tummy muscles** pulled in throughout the move. Repeat 25 times.

EXERCISE FOR **FITNESS-PHOBES**

If pounding the treadmill or pumping iron in the gym is your idea of torture or if you're just too busy to get there, take heart: many everyday activities can burn calories and help **tone** your body. So, if you put together enough short bursts of activity during the course of an ordinary day, you won't even need to drag yourself to the gym.

The key to success is putting in that extra bit of effort. In other words, make sure you move with vigour and get up a bit of a sweat for about 30 minutes every day.

Still don't believe it? Read on and you'll discover how you can make **ordinary things** such as shopping, sex and housework count towards getting you in shape.

HOUSEWORK

According to research at the Medical College of Wisconsin, Milwaukee, cleaning, polishing and vacuuming can be as good at **fighting flab** as a workout at the gym. So, if you don't get the chance to work out very often, view housework as offering you the perfect opportunity to burn calories and get your heart and lungs in good shape. Put some time and real energy into household tasks and you'll get a double payoff: a fitter body and a neater home.

Calories burned in 60 minutes:
- ✪ Washing the car 330
- ✪ Cleaning windows 170
- ✪ Making the bed 120
- ✪ Ironing 105

★**TIP** Most cleaning is great for toning your arm muscles, but help flatten that tummy by pulling it in as you work.

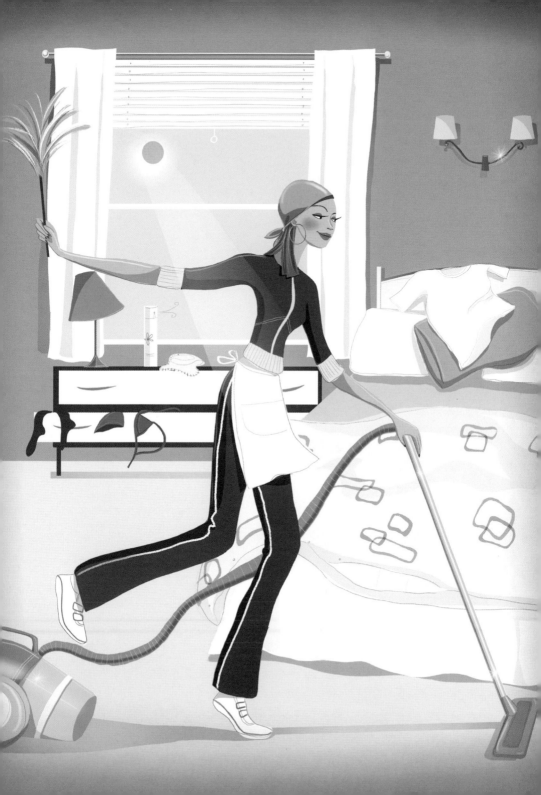

SHOPPING

It's the new aerobics! Walking fast and carrying bags of shopping can be an effective calorie burner and toner. Hotfoot it to the shops rather than driving or catching the bus to maximize these effects. Carrying heavy bags will also help **sculpt your arm muscles**, but make sure you carry an equal weight in each hand to keep things balanced and avoid back problems.

How to get more from your shopping workout:
* Use the stairs instead of the escalators in all the department stores you visit.
* Eat before you go – then you won't be tempted to gorge on sweets or chocolate along the way.
* If you're 'doing lunch' with a friend while you shop, don't wait until you're absolutely starving to stop and eat or you'll end up overeating. Also, plan to go somewhere that serves healthy, low-fat food.

GARDENING

Great news if you've got green fingers but hate the gym: gardening can reap the same benefits as a session on the treadmill. Raking leaves and cutting the lawn are two excellent choices. And as long as you **push yourself** hard enough to raise your heart rate and quicken your breathing, you'll be doing your body lots of good. Plus, you'll enjoy the benefits of stretching and strengthening your muscles. With this kind of workout, you also get plenty of fresh air and let go of a lot of stress and, of course, your plants will thrive along with you!

Calories burned in 60 minutes:
* Digging 300
* Raking leaves 200
* Weeding 200
* Mowing the lawn 150

SEX

Making love regularly is one of the best – and most enjoyable – ways to shift a few pounds: 30 minutes in the bedroom will burn around 150 calories. It'll also boost your circulation, throw your stress to the winds and **lift your mood**. And remember, the longer it lasts, the better the health benefits.

Even just kissing is good exercise, using lots of facial muscles, keeping them toned and helping to ward off wrinkles!

★**TIP** Choose a position in which you have to work harder if you want to maximize the amount of calories you burn – you on top, for example.

Six other ways to shape up without noticing

1 Chuck the remote – always getting up to change channels on the TV instead of using the remote control can burn 100–150 calories.
2 Don't send emails at work – walk over to your colleagues to discuss things with them.
3 Never take the lift (elevator) and always walk up escalators.
4 Make a point of using a toilet on a different floor at work and take the stairs to get there.
5 Buy a piece of fitness equipment and jump on it whenever you have a few minutes to spare. Even 5 minutes here and there will soon add up and psychologically spur you on.
6 Carry one bag at a time into the house when you're unloading shopping or rubbish from your car.

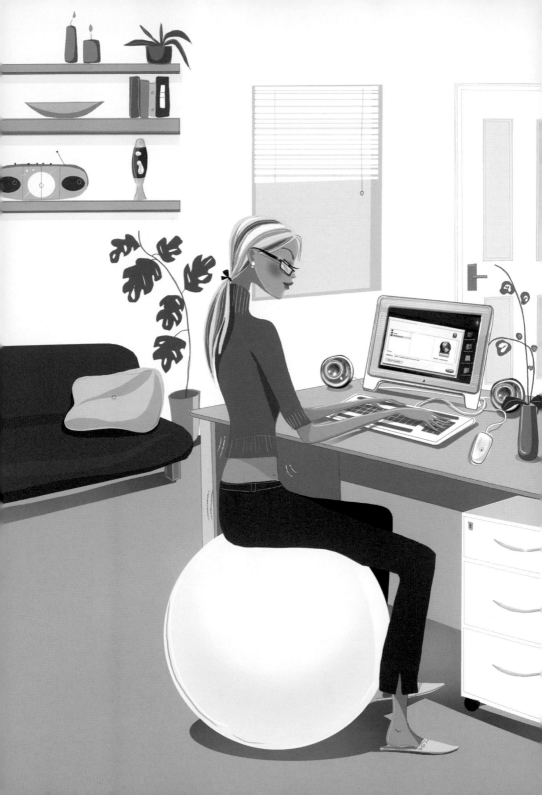

WORKOUT AT WORK

The deadlines are piling up; there are calls to be made and emails to send, so you'll be lucky if you even get time for a sandwich at lunch – a familiar story? There are always times when, despite the best intentions, you really are just **too busy** to hit the gym. Does this mean that your fitness regime has to go out the window, allowing the pounds to start piling on? Not if you apply a bit of lateral thinking.

There are plenty of potential exercise opportunities at the office and even a few moves that you can practise as you sit at your computer – without your boss realizing what you're doing!

HAVE A BALL

Buy an exercise ball and use it instead of a chair. Because sitting on it forces you to use **your 'core' muscles**, this simple substitution will strengthen your abs and lower back muscles and improve your overall posture – and without you even trying.

GET UP

Set your watch or phone alarm to **beep every hour** (but turn down the volume to avoid annoying all your colleagues!). This will remind you to get up and move around throughout the day. Even a walk to the toilet or a trip to the coffee machine will burn a few calories, stretch out your muscles and help to relieve stress.

STEP TO IT

Buy yourself a pedometer (available from most good fitness shops). This is a small, discreet gadget that can be clipped onto your waistband, which will keep track of exactly how many steps you take per day. This will encourage you to walk at every opportunity to clock up a high total – and afterwards to beat your own 'personal best'. To boost fitness levels and **burn maximum calories** you need to aim to take 6,000–10,000 steps each day.

DON'T MAKE IT **EASY** ON YOURSELF

Even though it's tempting if you're busy, get out of the habit of always going for the lazy option. Walk the flight of stairs up to the department you're sending a memo to instead of using the internal mail. The exercise will also help to wake you up if you're suffering from an afternoon energy slump.

MAKE LIKE **MADONNA!**

Get a headset for your office phone so that you can walk around while you're talking. If this isn't possible, remember to get up and **take a break** between calls to stretch your arms and avoid neck strain. Plus, just getting out of your chair will burn some calories.

TAKE A **STROLL**

Instead of having a coffee break, go for a '**walk break**' around the office. And at lunchtime, instead of sitting for the full hour to eat, devote some of your break to getting outside and taking a walk.

MAKE YOUR OFFICE **FITNESS-FRIENDLY**

Research has shown that exercise can both relieve stress and make workers more productive, so if your office, as some do, has an unspoken policy that its employees work through lunch, change it! You should not be expected to work during this period, so get together with co-workers and start taking your **whole lunch hour** – even if you're really strapped for time, at least try to go for a 15-minute walk outside. Better still, encourage your colleagues to help you persuade the boss to set up a deal with a local gym offering cut-price membership to company employees so that you can spend the whole hour there.

Five exercises you can do at your desk
1 Ab cruncher

Tighten your abs while you're sitting at your desk. When you exhale, pull in your stomach, pushing the air out. Pull it in tightly and quickly, then let it out naturally as you breathe air back into your lungs. Repeat 10 times.

2 Back strengthener

Sit upright on your chair with your feet flat on the floor. Relax your whole body as you press your abdomen back towards your spine and exhale. Pull your tailbone forwards and up and let your lower back drop down towards the floor. Hold for 5 seconds, then release your abdominals. Repeat 10 times.

3 Neck stretcher

As you sit in your chair, arch your back and turn your head to the right. Inhale and exhale. Then turn your head to the left, still arching your back, and inhale and exhale again. Finally, turn your head to the centre. Repeat the whole pattern 10 times.

4 Arm soother

Stand up, about two feet from your desk. Place your hands on the desk and keep them straight. Then, bend your arms and let your chin drop to within an inch or so of the desk. Straighten your arms again, straightening up your upper body. Then bend again, remembering to inhale and exhale throughout as you repeat the exercise 10 times.

5 Leg toner

Extend one leg out in front of you as you sit at your desk. Lift it a few inches off the floor and hold for approximately 20–30 seconds (lowering your leg more quickly if it starts to quiver). Then repeat the move with the other leg. As your legs get stronger, you can continue to tone your leg muscles – or push them a bit more even – by adding ankle weights. Repeat 10 times.

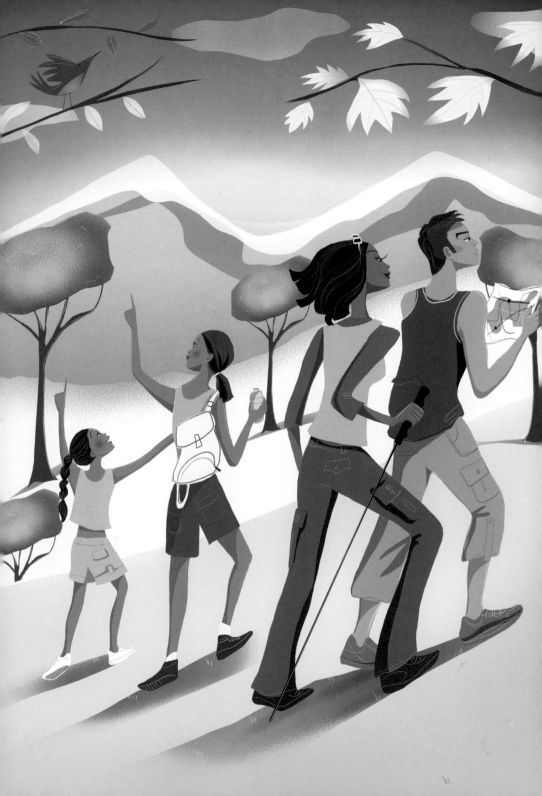

FAMILY FITNESS

If you're a mother juggling children, work and a social life, exercise can be pretty low on your agenda, which makes getting in shape especially difficult.

The answer is to incorporate family walks, swimming, games etc. into your lifestyle in such a way that they don't feel like a chore or take up lots of time. They'll still manage to boost the **fitness levels** of both you and your kids.

HOW TO **GET STARTED**

Plan regular exercise slots for the week ahead. Then take it in turns to choose what activity the family is going to do as a group each week. It could be family walks, swimming, cycling, **playing games** etc. Initially, it might seem difficult to find time for family fitness, but it won't be long before that Saturday morning trip to the pool or a Tuesday night walk to the park becomes second nature. And, according to fitness experts, when exercise becomes a habit you'll really start to reap the benefits.

TAKE A **HIKE**

Get the whole family together for a walk in the **local park**, forest or nature reserve. Take a healthy picnic to enjoy as a halfway reward.

★**TIP** A sibling, cousin or other family member can make the ideal personal trainer. Not only will you get quality time with someone you care about, but because they know you they can push you just when you need it.

HEAD FOR THE **PARK**

Play tag or throw a Frisbee – as long as you're moving about **vigorously** enough to get your heart beating faster, you're getting a good workout.

GO ON, DIVE IN

Find a pool that has a wave machine and water chutes. Your kids will be more inclined to stay in the water for longer if they're having fun, and that will allow you and your partner to swim more lengths.

BECOME A **SKATER**

Take your kids ice-skating or rollerblading; it's just as much **fun** for grown-ups and it's great for toning hard-to-reach areas too – your bottom and outer thighs, for instance.

★**TIP** Never skated before? Sign up for a couple of lessons from a seasoned instructor to learn the basics.

GET ON **YOUR BIKE**

Ride bikes together. If you have children who are learning to ride a bicycle, jog alongside while they ride.

Fitting in fitness

If your children are too young to workout with you, utilize the time when they are being looked after by friends or grandparents to exercise. And if you don't want to do it alone, getting together with other mothers to go for a run or to a yoga class while the kids are at playgroup is ideal.

HOLIDAY FITNESS

HOW TO USE YOUR VACATION TO GET FIT
BUT STILL HAVE FUN

The very idea of working out on vacation might leave you colder than the ice in your strawberry daiquiri but, equally, returning with an extra 2.5 kg (5 lb) to go with your new tan is probably the last thing you want. The key to avoiding this scenario is to find ways to exercise that require so **little effort** that it doesn't feel like a workout, activities that are such fun that you won't even notice you're exercising! The good news is that just swimming in the sea and playing a few beach games will get you burning more calories than you do back home.

POWER-WALK

If you go for a fast walk on the beach as the sun comes up or sets, or walk briskly from sight to sight while you're out culture-vulturing, you'll tone your legs and bum, so that you can enjoy that ice cream guilt-free.

Calories burned per 60 minutes: 350

SWIMMING

Tempting though it is to lie on your sun lounger, sipping cocktails all day, diving into the pool for a few lengths or into the sea, even for a short time, is a great way to tone your arms and legs simultaneously.

Calories burned per 60 minutes: 400

WATER SPORTS

If you're feeling more adventurous, try water-skiing or **windsurfing**. They'll give your arms an amazing workout. Don't worry if you find it hard to stand up at first – all the getting up and into position burns lots of calories.

Calories burned per 60 minutes: 300

BEACH GAMES

Just throwing a Frisbee or ball with a partner or friend on the beach will give your upper arms and shoulders a great workout.

Calories burned per 60 minutes: 200

VOLLEYBALL

This game is so much fun! Although very energetic, it gets quite competitive, so you won't have time to feel tired! Plus, all that running and **jumping** is great for firming your lower body.

Calories burned per 60 minutes: 350

HORSE-RIDING

Start the day with an exhilarating ride along the beach and you'll burn enough calories to allow yourself to indulge in a big breakfast.

Calories burned per 60 minutes: 270

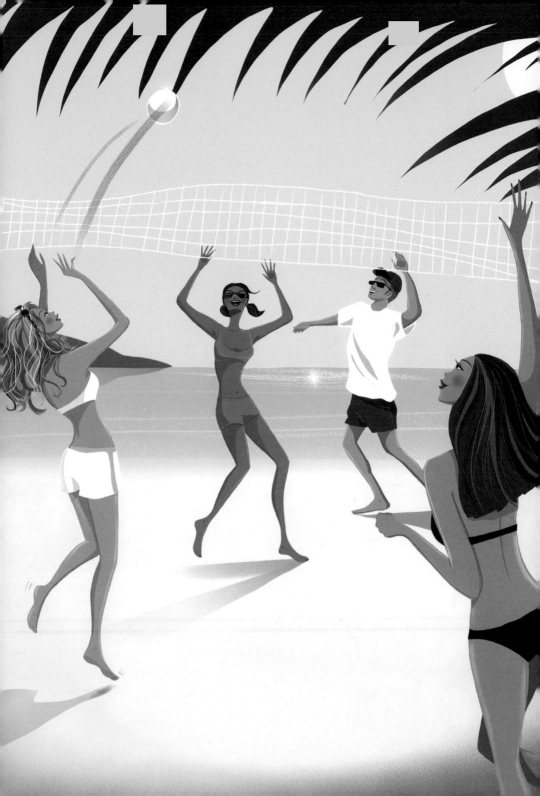

FIVE SNEAKY EXERCISE MOVES
THAT YOU CAN DO ANYWHERE

If all that still feels a bit energetic, try these during the day to keep you toned. They take no time at all and, best of all, you don't even have to stop sunbathing!

Tummy tucker – helps to flatten bulging bellies

Lie face down on your stomach with your head sitting on the back of your hands – even as you laze on your lilo. Then, gently but firmly, pull in your **abdominal muscles**, lifting your stomach up and away from the floor. Keep your bottom soft, your lower back straight and the rest of your body still. Hold your stomach muscles up for as long as you can, breathing normally throughout. Repeat 20 times.

Bum blitzer – lifts and tightens saggy bottoms

Easily done while you're waiting at the bar! Start by standing up straight with your tummy muscles pulled in. Then, as you breathe in, firmly pull in your bottom and pelvic floor muscles as tightly as you can and hold for a count of 20. **Breathe normally** throughout, but keep the muscles hard and tight. Then, exhale and gently release the muscles. Repeat 20 times.

Arm shaper – helps to tighten flabby arm muscles

An exercise for when you get up to go and buy a drink. Stand tall with your feet slightly wider than shoulder-width apart and your knees slightly bent. Hold your arms out to the side, parallel with the ground and with your palms facing forward. **Rotate your hands** and arms so that your palms face behind you, keeping your shoulders down. Stretch your arms back as far as possible. You should feel the stretch in the biceps and across your chest.

Waist whittler – for when you're lying on the beach

Here's one to trim your waist and hips and create greater definition. Lie on your back with your feet flat on the ground, your knees bent and your abdominal muscles pulled in tight. Hold your hands by your ears and, as you breathe out, slowly lift your head and shoulders off the floor to the count of three and pull your left shoulder towards your right knee. **Hold still** in this position, keeping your chin lifted up rather than pressed into your chest. Then, breathe in and lower yourself back to your starting position to the count of 3. Repeat 20 times on each side.

Thigh tightener – streamlines your outer thighs so they look slimmer in your bikini

An easy one to do on your sun lounger. Start by lying on your right side with your legs out straight, then stretch your right arm above your head so you're resting your head on your right arm. Then bend your left arm and place your palm on the lounger, in front of your chest. Next, lift your left leg a few inches and **point your toes** towards the sky, turning your leg out from the hip. Lift your right leg up to meet your left leg until your heels touch, hold for a count of 3 and then lower again. Repeat 20 times on each leg – or each time you change sides!

How to keep up the good work once you get back home

★ If you swam every morning on holiday, find a local pool where you can do the same.

★ Continue drinking plenty of mineral water. Not only will it keep you hydrated but, because the body often confuses thirst with hunger, it'll stop you overeating.

★ If the hotter holiday weather made you eat smaller portions of food throughout the day, then try to stick to that portion size on your return to cooler climes.

★ If you did your sightseeing on foot, you probably got lots of extra exercise. Apply this principle to your everyday life and ditch the car in favour of a stroll whenever you can.

★ If you enjoyed learning a new sport, such as water-skiing, scuba-diving or volleyball, resolve to make it your new hobby and find your nearest club as soon as you get back so that you can carry on with it.

BURN DOUBLE THE FAT
IN HALF THE TIME – INTERVAL TRAINING

If you're finding it hard to set aside gym time, you could try an abbreviated workout. It's possible to spend half the time working out and still reap the same **fat-burning** and body-toning benefits. The secret is to increase the intensity of your exercise to compensate for the reduction in time taken, a method that has the power to transform your body from flabby to fit in no time.

WHAT IS INTERVAL TRAINING?

Interval training is a method in which you alternate short peaks of exercise, when you're pushing yourself as hard as you can, with slower, gentler periods that give your body a chance to recover and allow you to get your breath back.

As well as increasing the amount of calories you burn during the actual workout, this way of exercising will also help you to **burn more calories** for the rest of the day. In fact, studies have shown that your metabolic rate will remain raised for up to 15 hours after interval training, compared with just 3 hours after normal exercise.

The fact that exercising like this actually turns your body into a more efficient fat-burning machine means that it's becoming a very popular way to exercise.

THE **SCIENCE BIT** – HOW IT WORKS

Your body burns different kinds of fuel after different kinds of exercise. During a steady workout you burn more fat, but as soon as you stop working out your body goes back to burning glucose (sugar). When you interval train, however, you **exercise more intensely**, which means that you use up your glucose stores more quickly, forcing your body to turn to your fat stores for energy during the rest of the day. As your body can't restock glucose straight away, you end up burning fat for longer after you've finished your workout.

HOW CAN I DO IT?

You can interval train doing any form of exercise, from swimming and running, to climbing the stairs. You simply have to mix bursts of high intensity with slower, recovery periods.

Five ways you can use **interval training** to halve your workout time

1 Swap a 40-minute run for 20 minutes of circuit training in which the pace goes up and down throughout.

2 Swap a 60-minute walk for 30 minutes on a treadmill walking up- and downhill.

3 Swap 40 minutes of breaststroke for 20 minutes of faster-paced front or back crawl – alternating between fast and slow lengths.

4 Swap a 6-mile cycle ride on flat country for a 3-mile cycle over hills.

5 Swap two 40-minute lunchtime weights sessions for 10 minutes every morning using heavier weights.

'IT AIN'T WHAT YOU DO,
IT'S THE WAY THAT YOU DO IT!'

Are you stuck in a rut with the same old workout that no longer seems to be helping? Maybe you've found that some moves leave you with an aching neck or troublesome knee joints? It's very easy to carry on, oblivious of the fact that you're actually doing your body harm while you think you're achieving the opposite.

There are some common mistakes that everyone tends to make at the gym, mistakes that can waste time, make your workout less effective, or put you at **risk of injury**. Here are some easy ways to correct them and ensure that you get optimum results from your exercise time.

SKIPPING THE WARM-UP

Even when you're in a hurry and don't have long to exercise, don't make the mistake of missing out on a warm-up. It's an **essential part** of any workout, because it gradually increases your heart rate, so that blood flows around the body and is directed to the muscles, making them more flexible and less prone to injury.

A warm-up need only last 5 minutes. Gentle jogging on the spot followed by a few stretches should do the trick, but try to make sure you **work the major muscles** of the body – including the calves, front and back of the thighs, shoulders, lower back and the bottom – as this will also increase the fluid in the joints so that they move more smoothly and easily.

NOT GETTING **EXPERT** ADVICE

If you're joining a gym it's vital that you have a proper **induction course**. One of the fitness trainers should take you around all the machines, explaining what they do and how to use them. And don't be afraid to ask questions if you're not sure about anything. Failing to get expert help could result in a lot of wasted time or – much worse – injury. Always consult your doctor, too, before beginning an exercise regime if you're pregnant or have any current injuries.

OVERDOING IT

Pushing yourself too hard will lead to burnout and injury. It'll also make the thought of working out so off-putting that you'll find yourself thinking up every excuse under the sun not to do it. This will make it almost impossible to establish any regular routine in the long run, so forget the **'pain is gain' theory**. Exercise doesn't have to be agony.

NOT PUTTING IN ENOUGH **OOMPH**

Failing to work up even a light sweat, on the other hand, won't do you much good either. If you want to shape up, exercise should be challenging, but not neck-breaking: working out at an intensity that still allows you to **hold a conversation** with the person next to you is enough to get great results.

EATING THE **WRONG FOODS** BEFORE EXERCISE

Some people don't eat before they workout because they believe that it's bad for them and will cause indigestion. In fact, a moderate-sized snack can improve your performance and many **top-class athletes** achieve better results when they snacked before – or even during – exercise. Think of all those tennis players who munch a banana mid-match, for instance.

A snack will restore and maintain blood-sugar levels, **preventing fatigue** and keeping energy supplies constant. It's best to go for something that contains carbohydrates, as they provide energy in an accessible form and are easily digested: a cereal bar, sandwich, banana or dried fruit eaten 30 minutes before your workout will provide an energy boost.

NOT DRINKING ENOUGH **WATER**

A recent study found that dehydrated people tend to workout for significantly shorter periods than those who drink plenty of water before and during exercise. Although most people know that maintaining hydration levels during exercise is important, the fact that the amount of water you drink has a huge effect on both the quality and quantity of your workouts is not so well known. Even a slight case of exercise-induced dehydration can cause your **aerobic capacity** to drop.

At the same time, bear in mind that overdoing it on the water-guzzling front can be just as bad for you, especially if you run long distances.

★**TIP** To work out your personal daily water prescription, divide your weight in pounds by two – the result is the number of fluid ounces of water your body needs a day.

NEVER **CHANGING** YOUR ROUTINE

Getting stuck in a fitness rut is bad on two counts. First, doing the same workout week in week out will gradually become easier, which means that you'll no longer be **challenging your body** – so your results will 'drop off', too. The other problem is that you'll soon get bored, which is when you're more likely to miss fitness sessions or give up completely. Avoid this by alternating between different types of exercise. Instead of doing three sessions in the gym each week, break them up: slot in a 40-minute stint in the pool instead of one of them, or, if you go running one day, try a yoga class the next time you exercise.

NO **TIME-OUT**

Some people view rest days as wasting time. In fact, they play a crucial part in your overall wellbeing. Rest allows your body to recuperate, so having a **day's break** in between fitness sessions means your muscle fibres have a chance to heal and regenerate. This gives your body the capacity to function properly, thereby making it possible for you to achieve your fitness goals safely.

BAD TECHNIQUE

If you're not getting results, or an exercise feels very uncomfortable, you're probably doing it incorrectly, so get expert advice from a **fitness instructor** at your local gym or buy a book or video that will explain visually how you should be doing it. For example, many people pull on their head and neck during sit-ups. This is certainly not the way to produce the washboard stomach you're craving and can injure your neck. Instead, place your fingertips just behind your ears to give light support, without the temptation to pull.

POOR **POSTURE**

If, as many people do, you spend your day in front of a computer, the chances are high that your shoulders will be used to slouching forwards and your spine will be rounded because most of your postural muscles have become lazy. Unless you consciously resolve to change it, this is the posture that you'll take into your workout, which will have **knock-on negative effects** there, too. The easy way to correct bad posture is to do a quick posture check before you start to exercise. Stand tall with your feet hip-width apart and your weight evenly distributed. Imagine your belly button is being pulled towards your spine and **keep your chest lifted**, your shoulders down and your back straight, breathing in and out deeply and regularly.

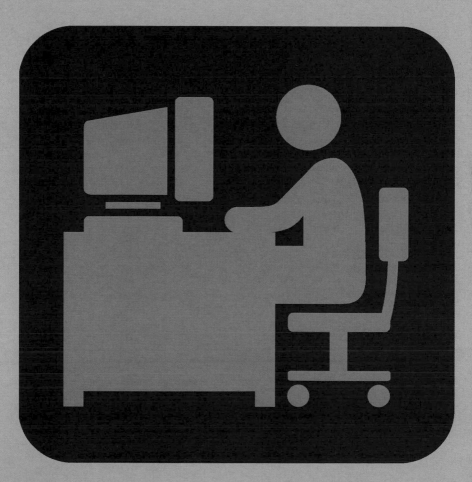

FUNKY NEW WAYS TO
KEEP FIT

If you find that the novelty of taking exercise wears off pretty quickly, it's vital to keep yourself physically and mentally **challenged**. One of the best ways to do this is to bombard yourself with new types of exercise. Nowadays there are so many fun, sexy or spiritual ways to workout on offer, being bored just isn't a viable excuse any more!

Here's a whistlestop tour of some of the latest, quirky ways to get in shape:

BODY COMBAT

This class has its roots in martial arts and combines moves and stances developed from a range of self-defence disciplines in an **adrenaline-pumping** routine. It could be described as aerobics with a martial-arts edge. Body combat teaches kicking and punching techniques that can then be put into a sequence to music. It also involves lots of shouting, so it's great for relieving stress! Physically, it's great for toning your legs and, because you're working your heart and lungs, you'll burn lots of calories, too.

Calories burned per 60-minute class: 400

THAI BOXING

This is one for the martial arts purist. It's a boxing class designed to exercise and discipline the mind as well as the body. The combination of arm and leg movements will **tone your limbs** and you'll also burn lots of calories and boost your general fitness levels, because it's so energetic. Plus, it should also improve your posture, coordination and flexibility.

Calories burned per 60-minute class: 450

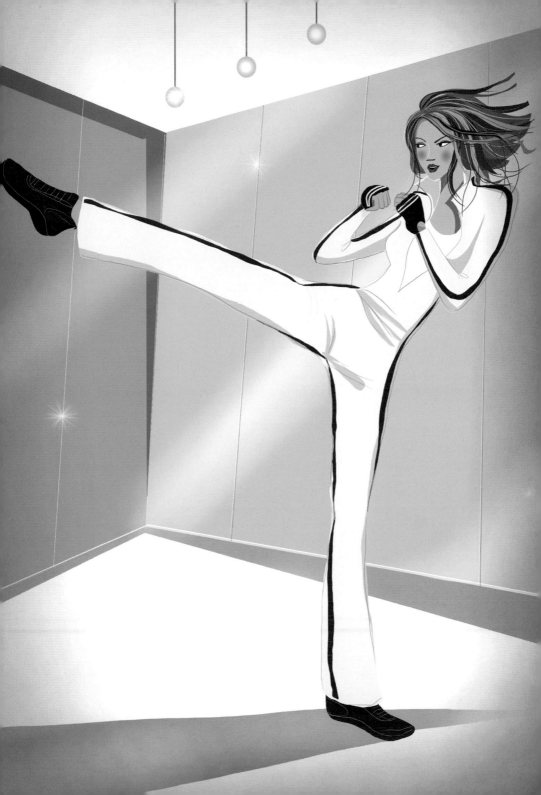

BALLET

Forget the tutu-wearing days of your childhood because ballet is fast becoming one of the trendiest ways to shape up – thanks, in no small part, to celebrity fans such as Sarah Jessica Parker. And frankly, no wonder it's so popular because doing ballet regularly will give you **fantastic posture** and long, lean muscles. The combination of stretches, lifts and exercises at the barre and on the floor works every last muscle in your body. This is the ultimate in overall toning.

Calories burned per 60-minute class: 300

AQUA JOGGING

Running is one of the best calorie-burning activities around, but pounding the pavement can wreak havoc with your joints, especially if you're already carrying a knee or ankle injury. Plus you may end up with 'jogger's jaw', a condition in which the facial muscles begin to sag. Jogging underwater may be the answer: the stress on your body is halved, but the workout is still effective. And it's perfect for firming hard-to-target areas such as thighs, bottoms and tums.

You'll need to stand waist-deep in water and jog slowly on the spot, using your arms as you would normally when you run, and increasing the pace when you get used to the **resistance** of the water. Holding weights or wearing a weighted belt will maximize the effectiveness of this activity.

Calories burned per 60-minute class: 600

SALSA

This hip-grinding, Latino dance is increasingly available as a fitness class at gyms. Not only is salsa very sexy, it's also great for boosting your confidence and teaching you how to **move to music**. As a form of workout, it's great for toning your calves, thighs, bottom and midriff. Lessons involve being taught the eight basic steps, and then how to combine them with simple spins and turns with your partner.

Calories burned per 60-minute class: 350–400

CIRCUS SKILLS

A class that teaches the skills of the big top, such as tightrope walking, stilts and trapeze, is the latest in **cutting-edge** fitness. You can even learn to ride a clown's unicycle! The emphasis is on **fun**; it promises improved balance, strength, speed, coordination and agility, and you'll end up with toned abdominal muscles, biceps, triceps and legs.

Calories burned per 60-minute class: about 300

★**TIP** Bored of the classes on offer at the gym? Check the advertisements in your local paper; they can be a great source for more unusual and exciting activities.

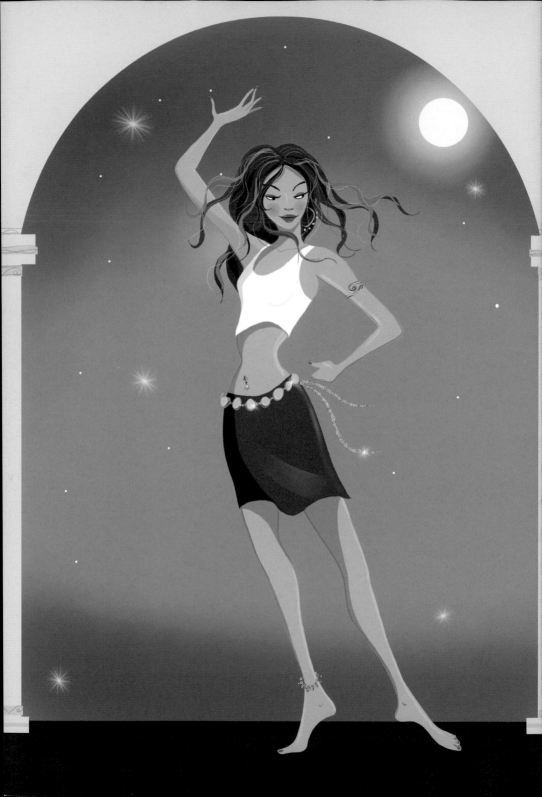

CREW CLASSES

This is basically a group rowing class designed to take the boredom out of rowing machines, much as spinning classes have given the good old exercise bike a new lease of life. You'll get a tough **cardiovascular workout** of 'virtual rowing' at varying speeds and intensities. Your arms will become ultra-toned and your leg muscles long and lean. You might like to alternate rowing with treadmill-running classes, which have a similar group emphasis, and which a number of gyms also offer.

Calories burned per 60-minute class: 400

BELLY DANCING

This Middle Eastern erotic style of dancing has been around for thousands of years, but its fitness benefits have only recently come into vogue. **Fashionable** it has become, however, and classes can now be found at many gyms. The flowing hip rolls of belly dancing use muscle groups in the abdomen, pelvis, spine and neck. During belly dancing, the joints and ligaments in your lower back and hips are put through a full range of gentle, repetitive movements. If these are done correctly, the pelvis is tilted forward, which should help to prevent lower back problems. Your arms and shoulders are also exercised, helping to keep them toned and slender.

Calories burned per 60-minute class: 390

FITNESS FACT FILES

It can be really difficult to decide what form of exercise is best for you, but these at-a-glance **summaries** of some of the most popular ways to get fit may help you make up your mind. Once you've weighed up the strengths and weaknesses of each and have decided how your body will benefit, shortlist those that target the areas and exercise goals that are high priority for you, and then pick one that will best suit you and your lifestyle.

RUNNING
What is it?

You see so many people pounding the pavement at lunch or after work and they make it look easy. Many who try running, however, simply end up out of breath and with some nasty blisters for their efforts. But despite its apparent difficulty, running has some pretty **powerful benefits**.

What's it good for?

Running is one of the most effective types of cardiovascular fitness training. You will get fit in a very short space of time, just by running 30 minutes a day, four days a week. It's a fantastic way to **lose weight**. In fact, few activities burn calories more quickly – just think of all the ultra-slim long-distance runners. It's also a very flexible method of keeping fit. You can run at your own pace, with or without company, and at whatever time of day suits you.

How do I get started?

Starting, then sticking with, a running programme doesn't have to be difficult. It's simply a matter of building up gradually and making sure that you take the time to warm up before, and cool down after, a run to **avoid injury**. Despite the hefty price tag, running shoes that fit well are a must if you want to avoid shin splints, blisters and sore muscles. Otherwise, apart from comfortable clothing, little else is required.

Calories burned per 30 minutes: 450

Tips for a **safe** running style

1 Keep your head level, avoid bouncing and lean forward slightly from the ankles, not the waist.

2 Keep your shoulders down and relaxed.

3 Strike the ground first with your heel and then roll to the ball of the foot, pushing off from the toes.

WALKING
What is it?

A great form of exercise – and one of the easiest. There's no need to go to the gym, join an exercise class, buy fancy clothes or expensive equipment and it can be done wherever you are.

What's it **good** for?

As well as keeping you in shape, a brisk walk every day can be more effective than drugs in treating mild to moderate **depression**. According to a 2001 report in the *British Journal of Sports Medicine*, just 30 minutes a day is enough to improve your mood significantly.

How do I **get started?**

All you need is a good pair of walking shoes. Start gradually if you want to avoid stiff or sore muscles and joints. It's a good idea to begin with a 15-minute programme. Think of your walk in three parts. Walk slowly for 5 minutes. **Increase your speed** for the next 5 minutes. Finally, to cool down, walk slowly again for 5 minutes. After several weeks, you can begin to walk faster and go further, and for longer periods of time too.

Try to walk at least three times a week, adding 2–3 minutes per week to the fast section of your walk. If you walk less than three times per week, though, increase your fast walk more slowly.

Calories burned per 30 minutes: 180

YOGA

What is **it?**

A 5,000-year-old practice that combines a series of bending/stretching postures with breathing techniques. It also involves learning **meditation** techniques to help you to explore your spiritual side.

What's it **good** for?

Not only will yoga improve your flexibility, strength and muscle tone, it's also great for helping you to relax and manage stress.

Research on cortisol (stress hormone) levels has found that yoga can help control pain by relieving stress and anxiety. It's also known to **reduce your heart rate** and slow your breathing. To be effective, yoga requires training and regular practice. You can find qualified instructors at gyms and yoga schools or you can learn about yoga through books and videos.

How do I **get started?**

When you first decide to look for a yoga class, you may be bewildered by the huge array of styles. Hatha yoga is perfect for beginners because it's designed to be **gentle** and is suitable for people of all ages and levels of fitness. Once you've got the hang of this style, you may want to **progress** to something like Ashtanga, also known as 'Power yoga'. Ashtanga yoga is fast and flowing, which will give you an aerobic workout as well as toning you. But be careful not to overdo it!

To avoid injury when you're doing yoga you need to know where your 'edge' is. This is the point where any less of a stretch wouldn't be a challenge, but anything more would be painful. You can linger at your edge, but don't go beyond it.

Calories burned per 30 minutes: 100

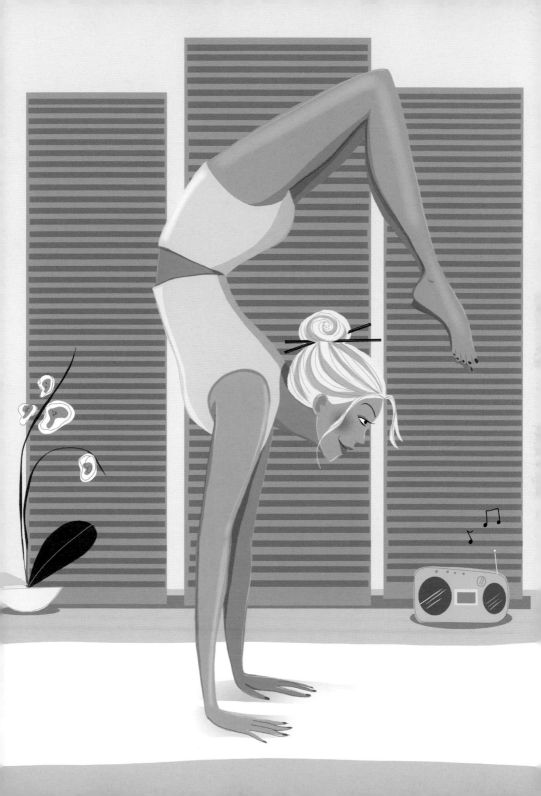

SWIMMING
What is it?

Easily one of the best forms of
exercise around as it promotes
strength, stamina and mobility,
resulting in all-round fitness.

What's it good for?

Regular swimming will boost your cardiovascular fitness,
muscular strength and **flexibility**, as well as helping to
reduce body fat. The resistance of water is perfect for
building the sort of firm, toned muscles you would
otherwise only get from weight training. One of the easiest
ways to create resistance in the water is to cup your hands
and push or pull the water away from you.

How do I get started?

Once you've decided to take the plunge, it's simply a
matter of finding a class that suits your needs. Check with
your **local sports centre** or gym. A good class should
include a warm-up, a period of cardiovascular exercise that
gradually increases and then decreases in intensity, and a
cool-down. Try to vary your strokes, to make sure you
work all the different muscle groups.

**Calories burned per 30 minutes: 200 for breaststroke,
nearly 300 for front crawl**

PILATES
What is it?

Pilates, named after its founder Joseph Pilates, is a total conditioning programme that works your body from the inside out by focusing on your 'core' muscles – those found in your stomach and back. It's also a **mind–body** exercise, which, like yoga, stresses the importance of correct breathing as you perform very precise body movements. Unlike yoga, however, the main focus of Pilates is exercise, while yoga is essentially a spiritual practice with physical wellbeing as one of the benefits.

What's it good for?

If you want to work your body to the core, exercising muscles you didn't even know you had, this is the workout for you. It's particularly good for **improving posture**, because it strengthens your lower back and abdomen. Plus, it will give you the trademark Pilates flat tummy and longer, leaner muscles all over your body.

How do I get started?

You do Pilates with special equipment, a mat, or both. A mat class is usually a **group class**, whereas equipment classes are more likely to be private. Contact your nearest gym, sports centre or Pilates studio to find out more. People often get frustrated and give up Pilates after a few classes because it can be difficult to get to grips with the initial movements without good tuition. So, don't sign up for a class with more than 15 people; otherwise, you may not get the attention you need from the instructor.

Calories burned per 30 minutes: 100

CYCLING
What is it?

If you don't like exercising indoors, cycling is a great way to workout. Running errands or just getting some fresh air by going for a bike ride with your friends or family can turn your much-dreaded exercise hour into a pleasure.

What's it good for?

Cycling isn't only fun, it's also a tough workout that really tones your legs, bottom and abs. Just make sure you wear a helmet. One of the best **family fitness** activities, cycling is also the one workout that allows you to cover some real distance. Most parks have marked-off bike trails these days so that you can ride without worrying about hitting anyone.

How do I get started?

You'll need to acquire a good bike, padded shorts to avoid a sore bottom and, most importantly, a safety helmet. When you're cycling **to get fit**, the first thing to do is to build up your endurance. Cycle a bit further each time until you can manage 30 minutes of constant pedalling; then incorporate some hills and bump up your speed.

When the weather gets bad in winter, it might be worth investing in an exercise bike or using one at your local gym if cycling is your main form of fitness training. That way you don't miss too many workouts because of treacherous conditions.

Calories burned per 30 minutes: 309

TENNIS

What is it?

Playing tennis is the classic way to spend a summer's day and is also an excellent workout that challenges your whole body.

What's it good for?

Just getting around the court involves a huge amount of running, making tennis a good cardiovascular workout. It's also good for improving **posture** and is a great arm, thigh and bottom toner. Working on your hand-to-eye coordination and your muscle strength will also help you deal with powerful returns.

How do I get started?

If you're a complete beginner, it's a good idea to arrange some **tennis lessons** with a professional to build your confidence and improve the overall quality of your game. Once you've got the hang of it, you can either enlist a friend as a playing partner or join a tennis club.

Calories burned per 30 minutes: 450

★**TIP** Don't just see tennis as a summer activity – make use of indoor courts so you can enjoy the game all year round.

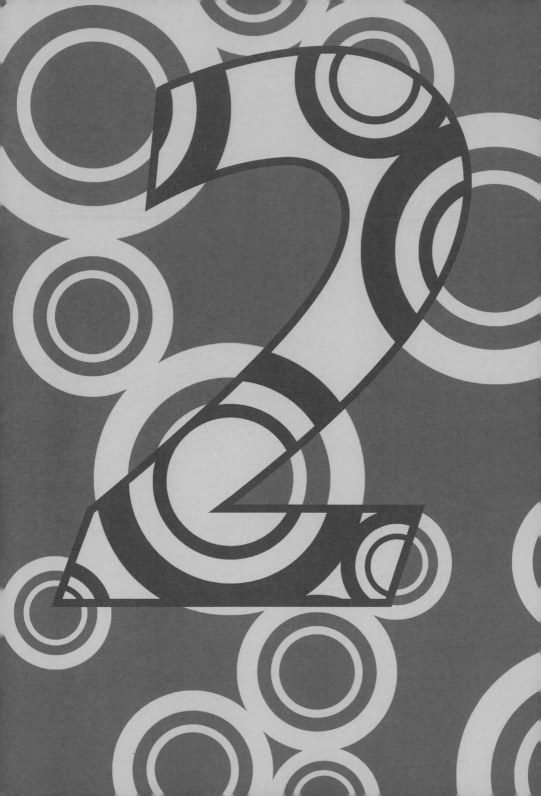

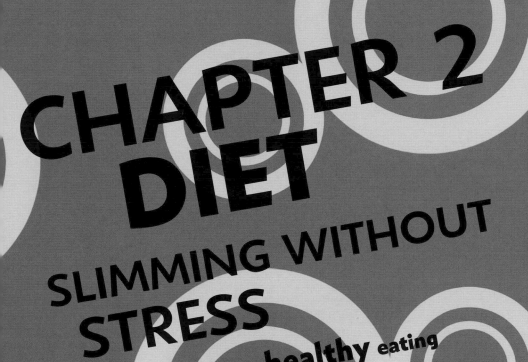

CHAPTER 2
DIET

SLIMMING WITHOUT STRESS

How to make healthy eating easy and **diet dilemmas** a thing of the past, whatever your **lifestyle.**

Losing weight and eating a **healthier** diet are at the top of every girl's wish list, but sticking with these good intentions, day in and day out, is not an easy task, especially when you're trying to juggle healthy food with a **busy lifestyle**. Eating on the run, work lunches and meals out with **friends** can all make dieting a real dilemma.

One of the main problems with dieting is unrealistic expectations – in other words, trying to **change** everything about your diet in one go and lose weight to boot is expecting too much. Even if you have iron **willpower**, the very act of depriving yourself has been found to lead to overeating. Rigidly banning certain

foods sets off a **natural** biological response: the desire to binge. Nutritionists say that the deprivation–binge cycle is **physiological** and **psychological**. So when you finally give in to what your body craves, you overeat.

The best way to begin is to make just a **few changes** at a time – for example, try only eating chocolate every other day instead of every day. This method will improve your **self-esteem** in the long run, as you are more likely to keep to manageable **goals** and won't give up so easily. And remember, as soon as you start to eat more healthily, you will find that you **look better**, feel better and have loads more energy.

SET **REALISTIC** GOALS

If you want to diet, decide how much weight you need to lose and work towards that goal realistically. Ideally, you should aim to lose about 1 kg (2 lb) a week. Although this may not sound like a lot, you're more likely to achieve permanent weight loss if you do it slowly. People who lose weight quickly on a crash diet tend to put it straight back on when they return to their normal eating habits. Changing your habits is more likely to make you keep the weight off long-term.

REWARD
YOURSELF

If you are being strict about counting calories, it's important to reward yourself every week. This will help strengthen your resolve to stick with the diet. Facials or manicures are great ways to treat yourself because they will make you **feel good** about yourself. If you can't afford to get them done professionally, ask some friends around and hold a **pamper party**. Get them to bring along some massage oils and nail varnishes and have a girls' night in.

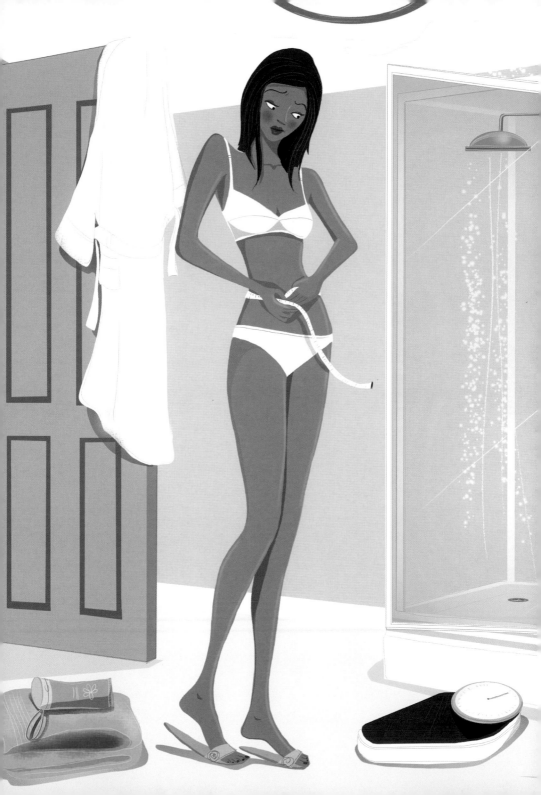

DON'T BE **TOO HARD** ON YOURSELF

If you eat too many choc-chip cookies one day or don't reach your 1 kg (2 lb) goal each week, don't beat yourself up. Everyone has days when they eat too many unhealthy foods. Instead, just decide to focus on healthy eating the following day. And if you aren't losing weight, persevere; fat takes a long time to work off and you'll get there in the end.

NEVER **SKIP** MEALS

The key to resisting the daily temptation of unhealthy food and keeping to a diet successfully is staving off hunger. The hungrier you feel, the more you will think about and crave food, and the more likely your resolve is to weaken. The trick here is to fill yourself up with plenty of high-fibre foods and to drink lots of water. Herbal tea is also excellent and a good alternative to your morning latte, which is packed with fat and calories.

★**TIP** To keep your metabolism ticking over between meals, nibble on healthy snacks, such as unsalted nuts, crudités and dried fruit.

SIX WAYS TO **KICK-START** A **HEALTHY**-EATING PLAN

Don't skip breakfast – it will make you feel hungry later on and slows your metabolism down.

Do eat snacks. Try not to let more than five hours go by without eating. Waiting too long can drain your energy and lead to overeating later.

Avoid carbonated drinks – most are packed with hidden calories and additives.

Aim to eat five servings of fruit and vegetables every day.

Buy pre-cut fruit and vegetables – this saves time on preparation and makes them easy to grab when you're in a hurry.

Take healthy snacks to work. Fruit, nuts and yogurt will help you overcome the temptation to hit the vending machine every afternoon.

Keep a **food diary**

Writing down everything you eat – and measuring the quantities – is a great way to become familiar with your eating habits. Studies show that most people vastly underestimate how much they eat, so seeing it written down in black and white can be a real eye-opener. Measuring your food enables you to become adept at assessing accurate portions, and keeping your portions under control. Keep a note of your feelings in the diary, too, as this can help to identify food triggers: for example, you might always crave chocolate when you've had a stressful day at work. If you're aware of this, you can then plan ahead and have some healthy snacks ready for times when you know you'll be under pressure.

WHAT NOT TO EAT

Food supplies us with calories, which the body turns into energy – this is then used up by physical activity. Put quite simply, if we eat more calories than we **burn off** with physical activity, we put on weight. Fat is a concentrated source of energy and just 1 gram provides 9 calories, more than double the calories of protein or carbohydrate. Like fat, sugar is a **dense energy source** packed with calories. Sugars are easily converted to glucose and can cause a rapid rise in blood **sugar levels**, giving you a quick burst of energy and a boost in mood. But if blood sugar rises too high, your body reacts by secreting insulin to clear the excess and this can result in an energy dip and hunger.

THE LOWDOWN ON FAT

Fat is an essential part of our diet but, in the Western world, most people eat far more than their bodies actually need. Eating too much fat will not only make you pile on the pounds but also increase your risk of heart disease, diabetes and certain cancers. On the other hand, cutting fat out of your diet completely is also dangerous and can lead to health problems. Fat is an essential nutrient that carries vitamins A, D, E and K and helps maintain healthy skin. It **insulates our bodies** from the cold and cushions our organs. Some fats help to make up important hormones that keep our body temperature and blood pressure regulated. The main point to remember is that all fats are not created equal – it's eating too much of the wrong type of fat that is harmful.

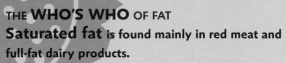

THE **WHO'S WHO** OF FAT
Saturated fat is found mainly in red meat and full-fat dairy products.

This is one of the baddies. The main problem with this type of fat is that it increases the level of 'bad' cholesterol in the blood, which can clog arteries and lead to heart problems. Your intake should be kept to a minimum. Choose lean cuts of meat and remove any fat before cooking, switch to low-fat (or nonfat) milk and cut down on butter.

Trans fat is found in hard margarine, cooking fats and processed baked goods.

Over the last couple of years more and more evidence is starting to emerge suggesting that this man-made fat may be even worse for your health than saturated fat. Trans fat increases 'bad' cholesterol and actually lowers the 'good' cholesterol that helps unclog arteries. Check food labels for trans fat – also known as hydrogenated oil – and try to avoid it as much as possible.

Polyunsaturated fat is found in corn, safflower and sunflower oils and also in sunflower margarine.

This is a fairly neutral fat. Although it lowers 'bad' cholesterol, it also lowers 'good' cholesterol as well. It's fine to include as part of a healthy diet, but not such a good choice as monounsaturated fat.

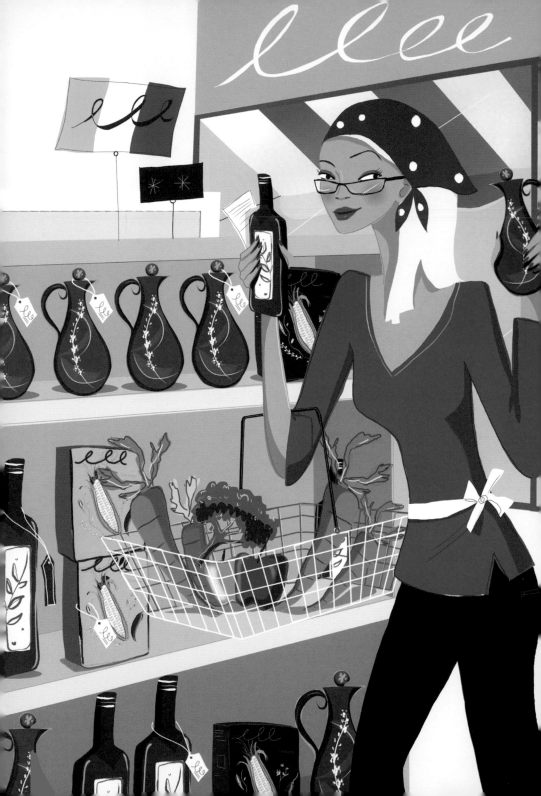

Monounsaturated fat

is found in olive oil, avocados and nuts.

This is the healthiest kind of fat you can eat and is actually good for you. It lowers 'bad' cholesterol and can raise levels of 'good' cholesterol. By switching to olive oil, you can protect yourself against heart disease and, as scientists now believe, help prevent bowel cancer.

Essential fatty acids

Omega-3 fatty acids are found in oily fish such as tuna, sardines and salmon. They help prevent blood clots forming and protect the heart. Omega-6 fatty acids are found in linseed oil and green leafy vegetables. They help boost the immune system.

Most of us get enough Omega 6 from our diet, but not enough Omega 3. To combat this, try to eat one or two portions of oily fish per week.

EASY WAYS TO EAT LESS FAT

- Always choose skimmed (nonfat or 1 per cent) or semi-skimmed (2 per cent) milk. Semi-skimmed has half the fat of full-fat (whole) milk, but the same amount of calcium and protein.
- Use an olive oil spread in place of butter.
- Substitute low-fat (nonfat) yogurt or crème fraiche for cream.
- Switch to half-fat cheese or eat smaller portions of stronger-flavoured cheese, which will give you a high taste factor for the calories.
- Make your own salad dressing with olive oil, lemon juice and balsamic vinegar instead of using mayonnaise or creamy ready-made dressings.
- Snack on nuts or dried fruit rather than crisps and biscuits (potato chips and cookies).
- Have fresh or baked fruit for dessert rather than cakes or pies.
- Microwave, steam, boil or grill (broil) rather than roast or fry.
- Reduce the amount of fatty meats, such as sausages and beef, that you eat.
- Eat pastry goods, such as croissants, in moderation; they contain a lot of saturated fat.
- Measure oil for cooking with a spoon, rather than pouring it from the bottle.

Watch out for low-fat foods

Products that are labelled 'low fat' are often loaded with other 'baddies' – E numbers, calories and artificial sweeteners. They also contain few vitamins and minerals. Low fat doesn't mean no fat; you could still be consuming some very unhealthy food. For example, some fat-reduced sausages contain over 10 per cent fat, which is still very high. To claim that a product is 'low fat' it needs to be at least 25 per cent lower than the standard product. But these types of food are often high in fat in the first place, so the 'reduced fat' version can still have relatively high amounts of both fat and calories.

THE LOWDOWN ON SUGAR

Sugar makes food taste good, but it can be highly addictive and lead to weight gain. Sugar is pure calories; it doesn't contain any other **nutrients** and we don't even need it for energy – we get enough energy from the other food we eat. The high calorie content of sugar is why too much of it can make you pile on weight. **Cutting back** on sugary treats and not adding sugar to food are the easiest ways to reduce calories without losing nutrients. To make matters worse, many sugary foods, such as cakes and chocolate, are also high in fat. Always check food ingredients for hidden sources of sugar, such as glucose, dextrose, fructose, honey and syrup.

FIVE SIMPLE WAYS TO CUT DOWN ON SUGAR

Drink low-calorie beverages.

Get used to drinking tea and coffee without sugar – try cutting it down a little at a time.

Spread jam, marmalade and honey more thinly on bread and toast.

Try halving the sugar you use in recipes.

Choose cereals that aren't coated with sugar or contain lots of added sugar.

WHAT A **HEALTHY DIET** SHOULD **CONTAIN**

OK, let's forget all the faddy, quick-fix diets for a moment and get back to basics: meat (protein), potatoes (carbohydrates) and vegetables. Studies show that back in the 1940s and 1950s, when meals were simpler and made up of the three main food groups, people **weighed less** and were healthier. A study by Professor Philip James, head of the think tank at the International Obesity Task Force, found that eight-year-olds currently consume on average 1,200 calories a day **MORE** than eight-year-olds did 60 years ago.

Today the reliance on ready-prepared meals and fast food has left many of us overweight and unhealthy. Most convenience foods are packed with fat, sugar and artificial additives; combine this with the trend for delicatessens, supermarkets and restaurants to super-size portions and it's no wonder the Western world is hurtling towards an obesity epidemic.

Preparing your own food, therefore, is the only way to control what you are eating. It doesn't have to take a long time; there are plenty of quick and easy ways to combine the following foods to make up your three daily meals.

PROTEIN

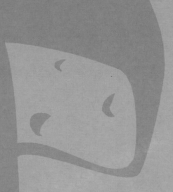

You should include protein with every meal; it helps fill you up and keeps your metabolism working at its peak. The healthiest sources of protein are lean red meat, chicken, turkey, game, fish, low-fat dairy products and eggs. Vegetarians should opt for nuts, beans, lentils and tofu.

CARBOHYDRATES

Like protein, some carbohydrates should be included with each meal because they provide fibre and much of the energy we need to get through the day. Avoid refined sources, such as white bread and rice, and aim for whole-grain varieties that have a low GI (Glycaemic Index). This means they are digested slowly, releasing sugar into the bloodstream over a long period, so keeping the release of insulin (the fat-storing hormone) under control.

FRUIT AND VEGETABLES

Aim for one portion of fruit with breakfast, two portions of vegetables with lunch and two again with dinner – this is an easy way to get your five recommended daily portions. Fresh, canned and frozen sources all count. According to a 2000 University of Illinois Department of Food Science and Human Nutrition analysis, canned fruits and vegetables, in most cases, are nutritionally equal to their fresh and frozen counterparts.

★**TIP** Plain, grilled meat and boiled vegetables are healthy but not exactly tantalizing for the tastebuds. Spice them up by adding a little pesto, garden herbs and lemon, or freshly chopped chilli, garlic or spring onions (scallions).

Cheat's guide to eating more fruit and vegetables

Although fruit and vegetables are rich sources of health-protecting vitamins and minerals, most of us don't eat enough of them. If the thought of eating five portions of fruit and vegetables a day fills you with horror, don't despair. Here are some easier ways to achieve your target:

Start the day with a smoothie
Using a blender or liquidizer, mix some soft fruit with low-fat milk. Try a banana, a handful of strawberries and some pineapple chunks – three delicious-tasting portions of fruit in one go!

Eat soup
Similarly, you can make or buy soup containing a variety of vegetables, such as carrots, peas, onions and celery. Again, you will get a lot of your daily vegetable quota in one easy meal.

Stock up your freezer
Perhaps surprisingly, frozen fruit and vegetables often contain more vitamins than their fresh counterparts. This is because they're frozen on the day they're actually picked, while fresh produce can take as much as two weeks to reach our supermarket shelves, thus losing some of its full vitamin content.

Cook carefully
Don't overcook vegetables or you'll leach out most of the vitamins and a lot of the taste. Use only a small amount of water or, even better, steam them using an electric steamer or one that can be put over a pan of boiling water. Alternatively, microwave them on high for a couple of minutes, again using only a little water.

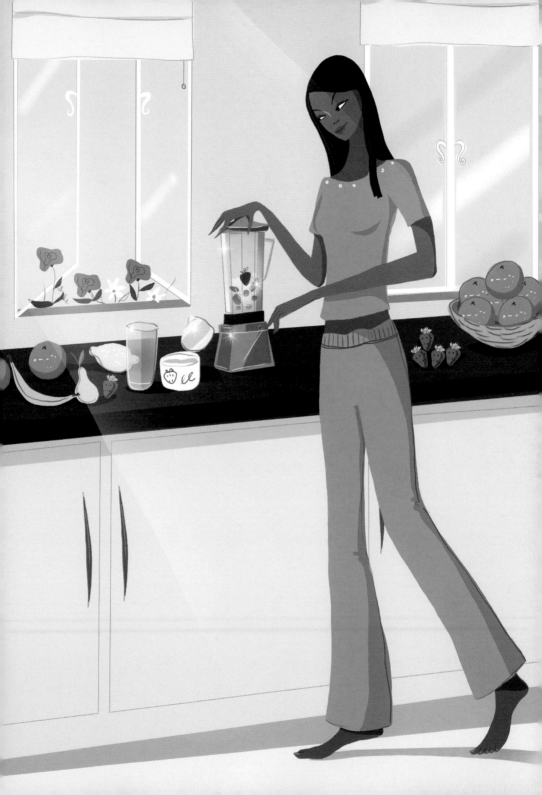

HEALTHY EATING
ON THE RUN

Forget about being a domestic goddess! Sometimes all you have the time and energy for is a speedy food fix, and you're not alone. In a 2001 UK Cathedral City Dairy survey, **over 65 per cent** of women said they found mealtimes a hassle, preferring to order a takeaway if possible. The fact is, these days our lifestyles are so busy that most of us don't have the **luxury of eating** all, or sometimes any, of our meals at home. Wander around any city at lunchtime and you'll see people rushing through the streets, munching hungrily on anything they can hold in one hand.

For most of us work takes up the majority of our time, then there are **friends to see**, the gym to visit and partners and family to spend time with. Fitting in eating healthily around all this activity is difficult, to say the least. But the problem with eating on the go is the **lack of quality** and **choice of food** on offer. Walk into your average store or snack bar and all you're faced with is high-fat and sugar-laden processed foods. So how can you stay healthy and trim when you're in a hurry? The trick is to become a whiz at creating nutritious but satisfying meals with the limited amount of time you have.

THINK AHEAD

Any diet can run into trouble if you wait until you're starving before you eat, and who's going to win when you come face-to-face with a co-worker's birthday cake mid-afternoon? A little planning goes a long way – if you know you're going to be stuck in a meeting all afternoon, take along something you can eat quickly and discreetly to keep your blood sugar from crashing and to keep your cravings at bay.

MAKE THE MOST OF LEFTOVERS

If you have a microwave at your office, pasta dishes and casseroles can be taken to work the following day in a plastic container and reheated for lunch. Alternatively, toss leftover rice or pasta in vinaigrette and add it to a green salad.

JUICE IT

Hit your nearest juice bar for an energizing fresh-fruit concoction – you can often choose the ingredients that go into it. If you have a kitchen at work, take in a hand-held blender and process chopped fruit and plain yogurt together to make a healthy, low-fat smoothie.

WRAP IT UP

For a portable meal that you can eat in the car or on the train, wrap up small pieces of chicken or fish in a lettuce leaf or small pitta bread. Throw in a few vegetables or chunks of apple and you've got a nutritious mini-meal.

TAKE A TRAVEL KIT

The key is finding healthy foods that travel well. Good choices include cottage cheese, yogurt, celery, peppers, carrots and apples. Make your own 'trail mix' of nuts and dried fruit and take it to work with you.

MAKE A LIST

Think of as many healthy snack combinations as you can – some fresh and some longer lasting – and stock up on all the ingredients you need when you do your weekly shop. This way you'll always have a variety of suitable nutritious options when that urge to snack strikes.

Six speedy low-fat suppers

Here are meals you can knock up in minutes using ingredients from the storecupboard and freezer.

1 Miso soup from a packet, with ramen noodles.
2 Vegetable soup with a wholegrain roll.
3 Baked potato with tuna and red peppers.
4 Frozen stir-fry mix and rice cooked in a wok.
5 Mixed canned bean salad with salad leaves.
6 Hummus made from canned chickpeas and lemon juice, with celery and carrot crudités.

HEALTHY SANDWICH OPTIONS

Grabbing a sandwich on the go? Sandwiches can range from the ultra-healthy to the downright sinful and that doesn't just apply to the ingredients inside them. We all know we should avoid fillings that are high in mayonnaise and butter, but did you know that the kind of bread you choose also matters? So, use your loaf and go for the healthiest variety to save calories and fat.

AT THE SANDWICH BAR:

SWAP
White bread

This popular bread is made from refined white flour that has been stripped of its fibre and nutrients for refining; and then fortified with the B vitamins (thiamin, niacin) and the minerals iron and calcium. It provides very little fibre, and also has a high Glycaemic Index, which means it releases sugar very quickly into the bloodstream, leading to energy dips and hunger pangs.

One slice contains: 79 calories and 1 g fat

FOR
Wholemeal (wholewheat)

This is made with flour that's ground from the whole grain, thus retaining the outer husk that's packed with fibre, and also the wheatgerm, which is high in B complex vitamins. Make sure the bread is not just 'brown' bread, which could be white bread that's been dyed!

One slice contains: 75 calories and 0.9 g fat

AT THE ITALIAN DELI:
SWAP
Focaccia

This Italian rustic bread is brushed liberally with olive oil and sprinkled with salt, making it fairly high in fat and sodium. Herbs such as rosemary and sun-dried tomatoes are often added for extra flavour.

One slice contains: 80 calories and 2.4 g fat

FOR
Ciabatta

A traditional Italian loaf, made with olive oil and with a lighter texture than ordinary white bread. It's made using white flour, so it doesn't contain much fibre, but it is a healthier choice than focaccia because it contains much less fat.

One slice contains: 73 calories and 1 g fat

★**TIP** Choose low-fat, high-flavour Italian fillings for your sandwiches, such as roasted vegetables and sun-dried tomatoes, but steer clear of Gorgonzola and other fattening cheeses.

AT THE MARKET:
SWAP
Naan bread

These Indian flatbreads contain clarified butter (ghee), making them much higher in fat than other types of bread. They are also often filled with nuts or meat, pushing the calorie content up even higher. They are best kept as an occasional treat.

One medium naan contains: 445 calories and 12 g fat

FOR
Wholemeal (wholewheat) pitta bread

Also known as 'pocket bread', pittas are traditional Mediterranean yeast-free flatbreads that can be stuffed with a variety of ingredients to make a sandwich. They have a similar nutritional content to ordinary white bread (see page 103) but the wholemeal variety is rich in fibre.

One medium pitta contains: 200 calories and 1g of fat

LOW-FAT **LUNCH BOXES**

Taking your own lunch to work has a dual benefit: you can **control what you eat** and it saves you money, so you have more cash to buy those great shoes or that must-have beauty product you've got your eye on. On the downside, however, it does require a little **forward planning** during your weekly supermarket shop and in the mornings, but if you get into the habit of making your lunch before you go to bed, it will soon become second nature.

HEALTHY CHOICES

✿ Make sandwiches using interesting breads, such as seeded, rye or pumpernickel, and fill with mixed salad leaves and tomato. Or choose egg, mashed banana, tuna or chicken fillings.

✿ Use the previous night's leftovers to make up pasta or rice salads. Try mixing in green or red pepper, cucumber chunks, cold chicken, tuna or kidney beans.

✿ Fill a thermos flask with soup to take to work in the winter.

✿ Replace cakes or chocolate with yogurt or fromage frais.

✿ Try to include at least one piece of fruit and make it easy to eat: for example, chop an apple into four or segment an orange.

★**TIP** Use the time when you're waiting for the morning coffee to brew or your iron to heat up to make and pack up your lunch.

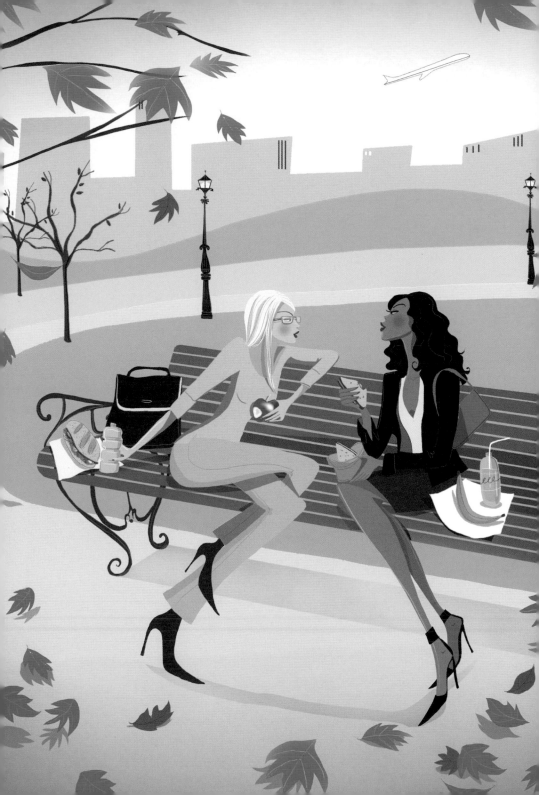

SNACK ATTACK

Eating regularly throughout the day is a good way to ward off feelings of sluggishness. Snacks keep your metabolism ticking over, which means you won't be starving when you come to eat your main meals – which is one cause of overeating. Also, if you're having a busy day and you manage to fit several snacks into your schedule, a missed lunch hour isn't such a disaster. What you choose to snack on, however, is crucial to the success of your diet, so here are a few strategies to help you enjoy those between-meal bites without guilt.

SAVOUR EVERY BITE

If you eat on the run, while you're working or even while you're watching television, you will find that your food is gone before you've even noticed it. Take time to sit down, turn off your computer if possible and **concentrate on enjoying** your snack. You'll eat it more slowly and find it far more satisfying.

THINK BEFORE YOU EAT

Surveys examining snacking habits in the workplace found that 61 per cent of snacks are eaten out of sheer boredom. So, before reaching for food, make sure you are genuinely hungry; if not, have a glass of water or go for a **fast-paced** walk.

CHOOSE **PROTEIN**

For long-lasting energy, have a **protein-rich snack**, such as small pieces of chicken or a handful of nuts. They will make you feel fuller for longer than starchy carbohydrates, such as bread, potatoes or pasta.

TIME IT WELL

Don't eat a snack just before a meal. In 2002, researchers at the University of Minnesota found that eating a snack half an hour before a meal means you will eat more food than if you snacked earlier. The reason for this is because your body sends out 'full' signals to the brain only after it's had time to **absorb the food**.

DON'T **DEPRIVE** YOURSELF

You should eat when you feel hungry. It's your body's way of telling you it needs fuel and it's always better to eat when you first get hungry than to binge later because you've starved yourself. Also, when you get over-hungry you're more likely to lose control and go for the less healthy option. The **'little and often'** rule helps avoid this.

HEALTHY **OPTIONS**

It's important to choose the right snacks because eating foods high in fat or sugar, such as chocolate bars or crisps (potato chips), between meals can increase your overall **calorie intake** really quickly.

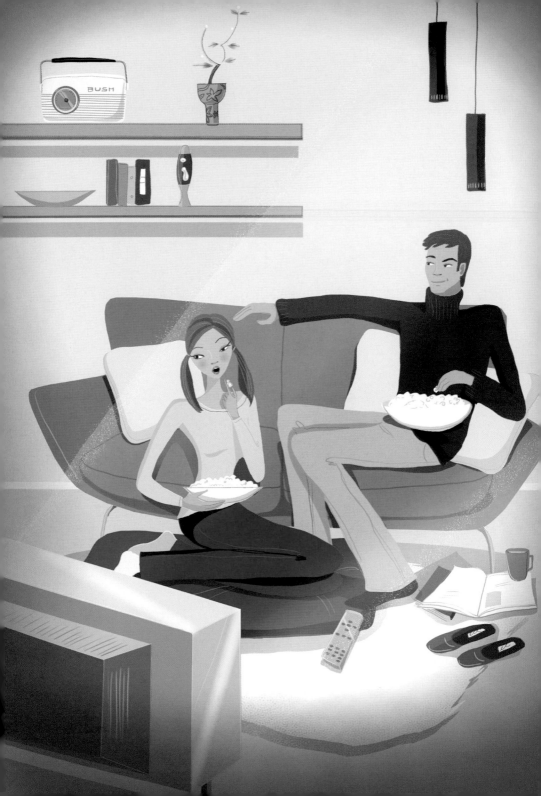

Wise snack **solutions**

★ A bowl of cereal with skimmed milk satisfies a craving for something sweet, but is much lower in sugar and fat and more nutritious than cakes or biscuits (cookies). Bran flakes or low-sugar muesli are good choices.

★ Plain air-popped popcorn sprinkled with paprika or a little Parmesan cheese tastes great, but contains very few calories.

★ Most supermarkets sell bags of ready-chopped raw vegetables – such as carrot or celery – which can be snacked on throughout the day.

★ If you're at home or have a microwave at work, baked beans on toast are a filling and nutritious way to keep mid-afternoon hunger pangs at bay.

★ Wholegrain crackers or rice cakes can be topped with a little peanut butter.

★ Easy-to-eat fresh fruit, such as bananas, apples and pears, boosts energy levels and provides plenty of nutrients.

★ A small handful of unsalted nuts will help to fill a gap and provides many essential minerals. A 2003 report from the *International Journal of Obesity* found that people who ate nuts as part of a healthy diet lost more weight than those who didn't.

TREAT YOURSELF

Diets that mean denying yourself any indulgences just don't work. You end up miserable and obsessively thinking about what you're not allowed, which can start a binge–guilt cycle or even make you give up on the diet completely. **Treating yourself** doesn't have to mean gorging on high-fat foods; try one of these delicious (almost) fat-free treats for all the satisfaction with only a fraction of the calories.

MERINGUE NEST WITH FRESH FRUIT AND CRÈME FRAÎCHE

Because meringue is made using only sugar and egg whites, it contains no fat. Neither does the fruit, so you can afford to top this treat up with a big dollop of reduced-fat crème fraîche. Choose **strawberries** and blueberries for your topping and you'll be boosting your intake of disease-fighting **antioxidants** at the same time.

HOT CHOCOLATE

There is nothing more comforting than a steaming mug of hot chocolate to warm you up and lift your spirits – especially on a cold **winter's day**. Normal drinking chocolate, however, has at least 140 calories and 4 g fat per cup. **Low-fat chocolate drinks**, on the other hand, contain only one-third of the calories per serving and virtually no fat, so will give you all the taste with none of the bad side effects.

TURKISH DELIGHT

We're talking the traditional variety here, not the chocolate-coated sort. Tell your friends and loved ones to buy you this exotic treat for special occasions, instead of the usual box of chocolates. It contains **no fat** and far fewer calories – just around 45 calories per piece – but it still feels indulgent and tastes **delicious**.

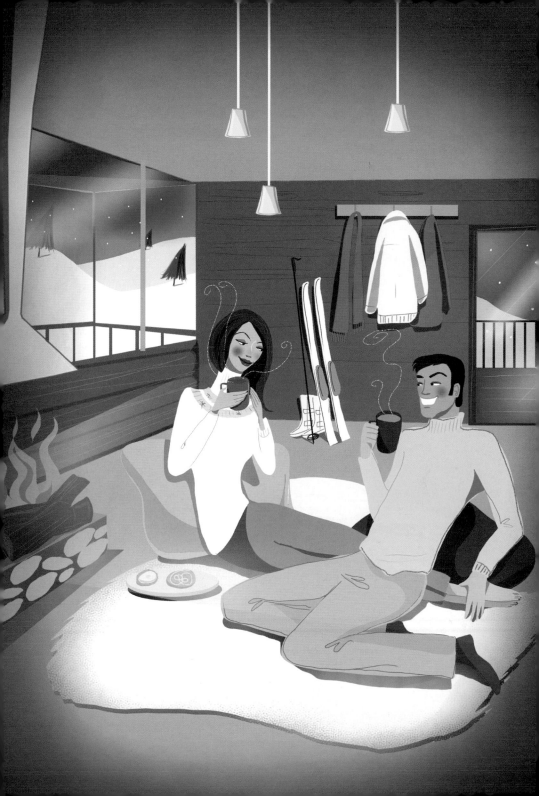

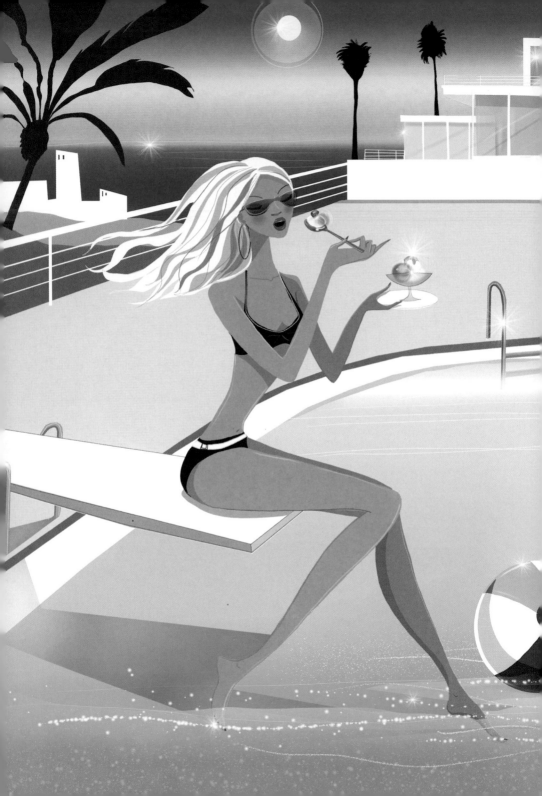

GELATINE

Revisit your childhood with a bowl of strawberry or lime jelly (jello). It tastes so good, you won't even notice that it's fat-free and if you choose the **sugar-free** variety you'll wipe out most of the calories, too. Toss some sliced fresh fruit into the mixture before it sets for an even fruitier **flavour** and more goodness.

A HANDFUL OF JELLYBEANS

These yummy sweets are completely fat-free, which makes them another perfect **replacement for chocolate**. What's more, they only contain 7 calories per bean – this means you can eat around 40 of them for the same amount of calories as in a small bar of chocolate.

TOASTED BAGEL WITH HONEY

Swap your morning Danish pastry for an unbuttered **wholemeal** (wholewheat) bagel with honey and you'll save calories – 250 calories and 1 g fat, compared with a whopping 445 calories and 21 g fat.

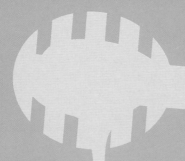

FRUIT SORBET

There's no getting away from it, ice cream is packed with fat. So, if you want to enjoy cool, **refreshing** sweetness, choose a sorbet or frozen fruit bar made from real fruit. Sorbets tend to be fat-free and **low calorie**, so you can enjoy your treat guilt-free while boosting your fruit intake at the same time.

WHAT'S YOUR FOOD
PERSONALITY?

Do you find it hard to stick to diets? Don't worry, you're not alone – studies show that a **shocking 90 per cent** of diets fail. But what makes dieting so difficult? Experts now believe they have the answer: it seems that what we eat and when we eat it may have more to do with our personality than genuine hunger. So, if you manage to eat healthily most of the time and only head straight for the bakery when you're stressed, you need a diet that's tailored to suit your 'food personality' in order to **lose weight successfully**. It makes sense: Everybody's different and so it's little wonder that a diet method that works brilliantly for one person could turn out to be a disaster for another. The right diet, however, should put your personality on your side, making weight loss easier and less stressful in the process.

Take this quiz to discover your food personality and learn which method of dieting is most likely to work for you.

Q1 WHY DO YOU THINK YOUR DIETS NORMALLY FAIL?

A My life is just too busy to plan meals carefully every day.

B I start off well, but the minute something goes wrong in my life my diet goes out the window.

C I'm OK on my own, but then my family and friends encourage me to lapse at mealtimes and social events.

D If the weight doesn't fall off immediately, I lose motivation.

Q2 WHICH STATEMENT BEST DESCRIBES YOUR ATTITUDE TO FOOD?

A I spend my life battling with it.

B I think of food as a treat, which can make me feel better when I'm down.

C I love eating! There's nothing better than enjoying good food together with good company.

D It's just fuel. I don't think about food that much really.

Q3 WHAT'S YOUR TYPICAL DAY'S FOOD? PICK THE ANSWER THAT BEST DESCRIBES WHAT YOU EAT EVERY DAY.

A I skip breakfast and sometimes lunch if I'm busy, and usually have a takeaway or microwave meal when I get home.

B I often miss breakfast, but usually have a good-size lunch and dinner to compensate.

C Breakfast, lunch and dinner with snacks in between.

D I don't have set meals, but snack throughout the day.

Q4 WHEN YOU'RE CRAVING SOMETHING, IS IT MORE LIKELY TO BE:

A Fast food, like a pizza or a burger.

B Something starchy and comforting like chips (french fries), bread or pasta.

C Something indulgent and rich like a scoop of ice cream or a piece of cake.

D Savoury foods such as meat or cheese.

Q5 HOW DOES STRESS AFFECT THE WAY YOU EAT?

A If I'm too busy, I skip meals and fill up on snacks.

B I tend to eat everything in sight as a way of helping me get through the busy time.

C It makes me lose my appetite; I can get to 5 pm before realizing I've hardly eaten since breakfast.

D It doesn't – I just carry on eating as I normally would.

Q6 IN GENERAL, WHAT DO YOU DO WITH YOUR FOOD AFTER YOU BEGIN TO FEEL FULL?

A Stop and leave what's left.

B I don't often feel full.

C Finish what's left – there's no sense in letting it go to waste!

D I finish it and often have a second helping, even if I'm not actually hungry.

Q7 HOW DO YOU PREFER TO DO THINGS?

A Alone.

B With one other person.

C In a big group.

D I enjoy both group and solo activities.

Q8 WHICH STATEMENT BEST DESCRIBES YOUR PERSONALITY?

A Generally happy, but prone to stress.

B Up one minute and then down the next.

C Sociable and fun-loving.

D I'm fairly relaxed and go with the flow most of the time.

MOSTLY 'A'S – THE **STRESSED-OUT** STUFFER

A busy schedule means that you tend to skip meals during the day, grabbing unhealthy snacks to keep you going and then having a huge evening meal to compensate. However, because you're often busy until late in the evening, phoning for a takeaway or microwaving a ready-meal is all you feel like doing when you finally get home.

Diet **downfall**

This type of eater often relies on sugary or fatty snacks instead of nutritious meals. Not only are such foods packed with calories but they also give just a short energy boost, which is soon followed by feelings of fatigue.

Most **effective** diet for you

Your lack of time makes online dieting ideal, as it's quick, easy and hassle-free. Most diet websites will tell you the daily calorie intake you need to stick to in order to reach your target weight, plus you can often enter everything you eat each day into a food calculator and monitor how you're doing.

Tips for success

✿ Try using some of the organization skills you employ at work to plan your meals better. Keep a box of whole-grain cereal or fresh fruit on your desk at the office and have a ready supply of healthy snacks, such as dried fruit and unsalted nuts, in your desk drawer.

✿ Learn that low-fat freshly cooked meals don't have to be time-consuming. Keep a bag of prepared veggies in the freezer for a quick stir-fry and stock up on tins of tomatoes with herbs for a speedy pasta sauce.

MOSTLY 'B'S – **COMFORT** EATER

You spend half your time being good
and the other half overindulging to
match the state of your emotions.
This sort of yo-yo dieting can slow
down your metabolism, making it
harder to shift weight in the long run.

Diet **downfall**

When things go wrong, you console
yourself with large quantities of your
favourite, typically high-fat, foods.

Most effective diet for **you**

You need a diet programme that will deal with the
emotional aspect of your weight problem. Organizations
such as Overeaters Anonymous can help if you think you
may have a food addiction.

Tips for **success**

✿ Next time you have a crisis, instead of reaching for
a cream cake, choose something unconnected with
food to make you feel better. Phone your most positive
friend for a pep talk or play your favourite uplifting
song at full volume.

✿ If you still crave that comforting sensation of being full,
include low-fat, high-fibre foods with every meal to
help keep you satisfied for longer. Good choices
include brown rice, wholewheat (wholemeal) pasta,
baked potatoes and couscous.

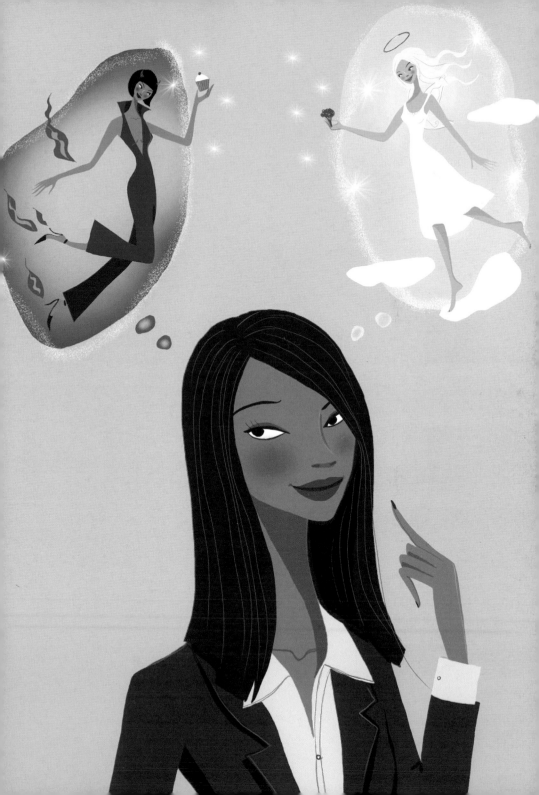

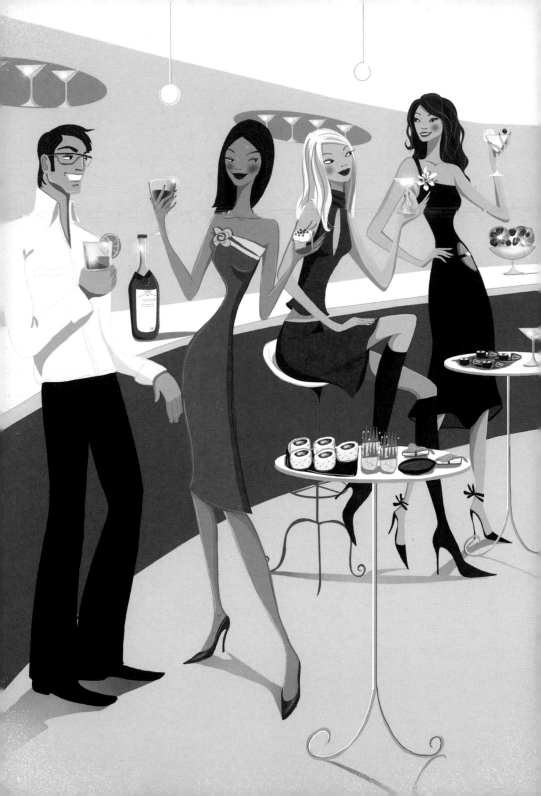

MOSTLY 'C'S – **SOCIAL** NIBBLER

You love eating and drinking in social situations, whether it's dinner parties or meals out with friends.

Diet **downfall**

Going without dessert when everyone else is having one makes you miserable; you'd rather skip breakfast and save the calories for later! However, several studies have found that people who eat breakfast every day are slimmer than those who miss it, as they are less likely to overeat later in the day.

Most **effective diet** for you

Your extrovert personality means you'll benefit from turning weight loss into a social event. A group-based diet method that involves regular meetings, such as Weight Watchers and other slimming clubs, will work best for you.

Tips for **success**

✿ Next time you have friends over for dinner, try making them a healthier meal. It's easy to swap low-fat cheeses for normal versions, reduced-fat crème fraîche for cream, and to use leaner cuts of meat without losing any of the taste.

✿ If you know you're going out for dinner in the evening, make sure you eat properly during the day. This way you won't be starving and will be less likely to overeat.

✿ If wine tends to be your downfall, try alternating each drink with a glass of sparkling water. It will halve the amount you drink and cut your chances of having a hangover the next morning!

MOSTLY 'D'S – MINDLESS MUNCHER

You're probably not that interested in food and see it as merely fuel. At the same time, you don't like waste and would rather clear your plate than throw anything away, so you sometimes overeat without realizing it.

Diet downfall

Because convenience and ease are your top priorities, the foods you eat tend to be high in calories and low in nutrients. As a result, you consume more calories than you think.

Most effective diet for you

Once you know the rules of healthy eating you are likely to be good at sticking to them. You'd benefit from learning more about nutrition, which will help you distinguish between good and bad food choices. It would also be worth seeing a registered dietician (your doctor may be able to refer you to one) who will work out a suitable diet plan for you.

Tips for success

✿ Remember, it's OK to throw food away if you're full. It's better than using your stomach as a garbage bin!

✿ Always sit down to eat rather than eating on the run.

✿ Avoid combining meals with other activities, such as watching TV. If you focus on what you're actually eating it's easier to register when your body is full.

DON'T TAKE AWAY MY **TAKEAWAY!**

After a busy day at work, a takeaway pizza or Chinese is the ultimate convenience meal. There are times when, no matter how many 'quick-fix' meals you have in your fridge or cupboard, you just don't feel like spending any time in the kitchen. All you want to do is sink onto the sofa with a **tasty takeout**. The only problem is that most types of takeaway food tend to be packed with hidden fat and calories. Some single dishes can even contain your entire fat content for the whole day! But, thankfully, watching your weight doesn't mean you have to forgo this luxury entirely. It's simply a case of knowing what to order and what to avoid the next time you put in a call to your local **food-delivery emporium**.

INDIAN
What to avoid
- Poppadums, samosas and onion bhajis, all of which are deep-fried and sky-high in calories.
- Cream-based curry sauces, such as korma and passanda

How to make it healthier
- Order dry-cooked tandoori dishes or tomato-based curries, such as rogan josh.
- Take advantage of the delicious vegetarian dishes on offer, such as lentil dhal, saag (spinach) and cauliflower.
- Go for boiled rice. It's much healthier than pilau rice, which is heavy on oil.
- Choose chapattis or roti bread – they're a much better bread choice than naan, which can be smothered in ghee (clarified butter).

★**TIP** With most curries you can cut out fat by tipping away the excess oil in the sauce before serving.

CHINESE
What to avoid
✿ Anything deep-fried will be packed with fat. That means ditching the prawn crackers, spring (egg) rolls, crispy Peking duck and seaweed.

How to make it healthier
✿ Choose soups, such as chicken and sweetcorn, wonton or hot and sour, that are much kinder to your waistline.
✿ Go for stir-fries that contain plenty of vegetables.
✿ Choose meat that isn't in batter. Good low-fat sauce choices include: black bean, teriyaki and soy sauce.
✿ Order lower-fat protein choices like chicken, shrimp or tofu.
✿ Have plain boiled rice rather than fried rice and share – rice portions are usually much too generous.

★TIP Eating with chopsticks will make your meal last longer because you'll eat smaller mouthfuls and so you'll feel that you've eaten more.

ITALIAN
What to avoid
✿ All the little extras – those calories soon add up. Ask yourself if you really need garlic bread, extra pepperoni or cheese, carbonated soda or ice cream.
✿ Super-sizing. Don't go for extra large just because it's better value for money.

How to make it healthier
✿ Share your pizza with friends and get a huge salad to go with it. This way everyone keeps an eye on the amount they're eating.
✿ Go for the deep-pan option. A thick-crust pizza contains a higher proportion of carbohydrate and a lower proportion of fat than a thin-crust version.
✿ Add extra vegetables or pineapple toppings. As well as getting a delicious treat, you'll be notching up your five portions of fruit and vegetables.

★TIP When you order, ask for half the normal amount of cheese and you'll slash your pizza's fat content.

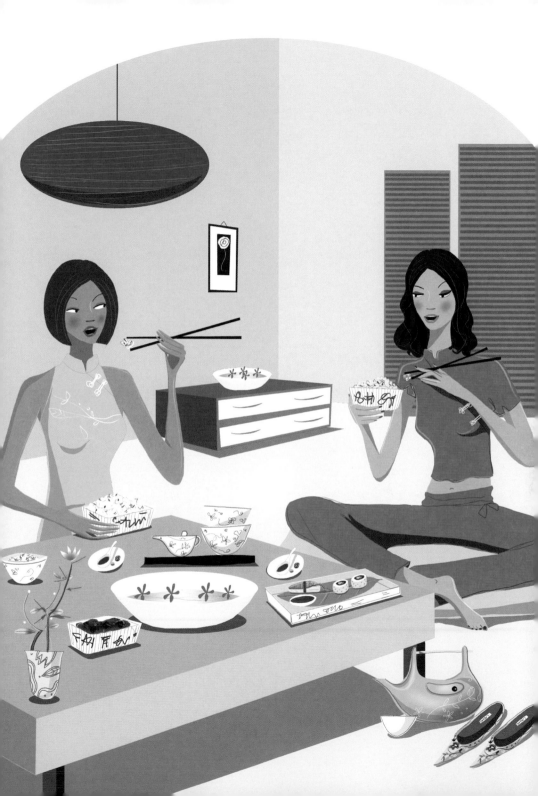

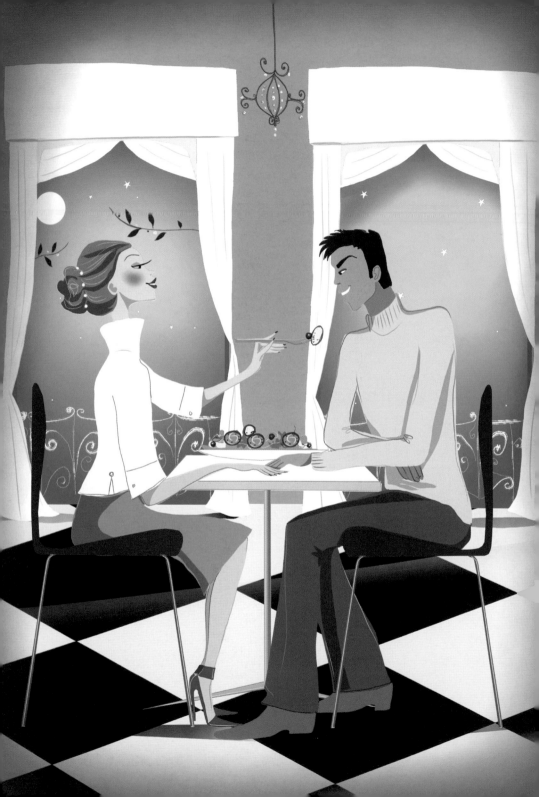

HOW TO **DIET-PROOF** A **MEAL OUT**

Eating in restaurants can be the downfall of even the most dedicated dieter. The meals often include too much fat, salt or sugar, and the portions are almost always larger than you would eat at home. By following a few simple rules, however, you can maintain your healthy eating plan and still enjoy a meal out with friends.

✿ Choose dishes that have been baked, grilled (broiled), poached or steamed. Avoid anything fried. Check with the waiter if you're not sure how something is cooked.

✿ Fill up with salads and extra portions of vegetables.

✿ If you know the restaurant you're eating at serves large portions, order a half size or a starter (appetizer) as your main course.

✿ Order sauce and dressing on the side. By doing this you can control the amount you eat and often you can manage with less while still enjoying the same taste.

✿ Sharing first courses and desserts with a partner or friend is a great idea as it means you get to taste something you want without overindulging.

★**TIP** Turn Japanese. It's one of the lowest fat cuisines around. Pick sushi, miso soup or stir-fried noodles with vegetables for tasty treats that won't derail your diet.

SALAD BAR
TRAFFIC LIGHTS

Salad bars in supermarkets and restaurants seem like a good way to eat more vegetables but, depending on what you choose, you may end up adding a lot of extra fat and calories to your meal. For example, many dishes are loaded with mayonnaise, which will soon turn your healthy meal into a fat-fest. Read on to discover which foods get the green light (meaning you can eat as much as you like), the amber light (foods have some health benefits but be careful not to overdo the portion size) and the red light (avoid at all costs).

GREEN LIGHT

Tomatoes

Rich in betacarotene, vitamins C and E, tomatoes are also a good source of lycopene – an antioxidant that has been found to help protect against cancer. They are, of course, also **low in calories**.

Rice and vegetable salad

A great, filling dish that's full of fibre and nutrients – particularly when it's made with brown rice. The vegetables the salad contains are **good sources of vitamins** and minerals, but steer clear of oily dressings as they can be packed with hidden fat.

Carrot and celery sticks

Both vegetables are low in calories so, as long as you're careful not to dip them into anything high fat, you can eat as much as you like. Celery is a good high-fibre choice and carrots contain betacarotene, which the body uses to make vitamin A. Betacarotene is also a powerful antioxidant, high intakes of which can help **reduce your risk of heart disease** and certain cancers.

Mixed lettuce leaves

Generally speaking, the darker the leaves the more nutrients they contain, such as vitamin C, folic acid and potassium. Again, watch out for oily salad dressings; try using **balsamic vinegar** or a squeeze of lemon juice to add flavour.

Tzatziki

If you can't resist dips, this is the one to go for. It's made with yogurt, rather than cream or oil, so it's much **lower in fat** but has all the taste and texture of some of the more unhealthy options, such as sour cream and chives or cheese dip.

AMBER LIGHT
Bean salad

Because they are very high in fibre, bean dishes are really filling. Pulses (legumes) are also a good **source of iron**, making them an important food for people who don't eat meat. If the beans are in an oily dressing, drain off as much as you can before transferring them to your plate.

Pasta salad

Although a good source of starchy carbohydrates, make sure you only choose dishes with a tomato- or **vinaigrette-based** sauce. Mayonnaise will make it high in fat and calories.

Cottage cheese

This is a rich source of protein **for vegetarians** and contains calcium, which is important for good bone health. You'll also find B vitamins, which help maintain a healthy nervous system, and it's low in fat. Choose cottage cheese rather than potato salad or coleslaw if you crave something creamy.

Toasted mixed seeds

Seeds are high in protein and contain good amounts of minerals, such as zinc, iron and selenium. Although they are quite high in fat, it's mainly monounsaturated fat, which is **good for the heart**. Toasting seeds brings out the flavour, so you'll only need a small sprinkling to enjoy the taste.

RED LIGHT
Tuna salad

Tuna contains lots of protein but unfortunately most salad bars use the variety canned in oil rather than in water, which **pushes up the fat content**. Choose only a small amount, as the mayonnaise bumps up the fat content.

Croutons

Keep walking! Croutons are usually cooked in either oil or butter, making them a very high-fat choice. Choose carrots or seeds if you want to add a **bit of crunch** to your salad.

Coleslaw

It might sound healthy with all that **carrot and cabbage**, but coleslaw includes lots of mayonnaise, making it a bad choice if you want to lose weight. If you can't resist, go for a very small amount and choose calorie-reduced varieties if available.

Potato salad

Unless it's the **low-fat variety**, potato salad is best avoided if you're watching your weight, as it is usually packed with mayonnaise.

Surviving summer barbecues

Don't let being on a diet ruin your summer. Barbecues are actually quite a healthy way to cook meat, because no fat is added. So choose wisely, and enjoy yourself along with everyone else.

★ Select low-calorie foods throughout the day, so you'll have extra calories to play with once you're there. Some people eat only fruit if they know they are going to be eating a bigger meal later in the day.

★ Make a firm mental note to only fill your plate once. Don't allow yourself to be persuaded otherwise.

★ Lay off the booze. Stick to water or sugar-free soft drinks. This saves on calories and will help you keep control over what you eat.

★ Choose chicken and fish where possible and remove any skin from the chicken.

★ If you can't resist sausages or burgers, buy the low-fat varieties if you are hosting the meal.

★ Fill a good half of your plate with green salad, but try eating it solo, without a dressing. Only choose a dressing if you're certain it's low in fat.

★ Help yourself to large portions of filling foods such as rice, pasta, potatoes and bread, but don't pile on the butter!

★ Avoid high-fat sauces that contain mayonnaise and oil – opt for lower-calorie alternatives like tomato ketchup or salsa.

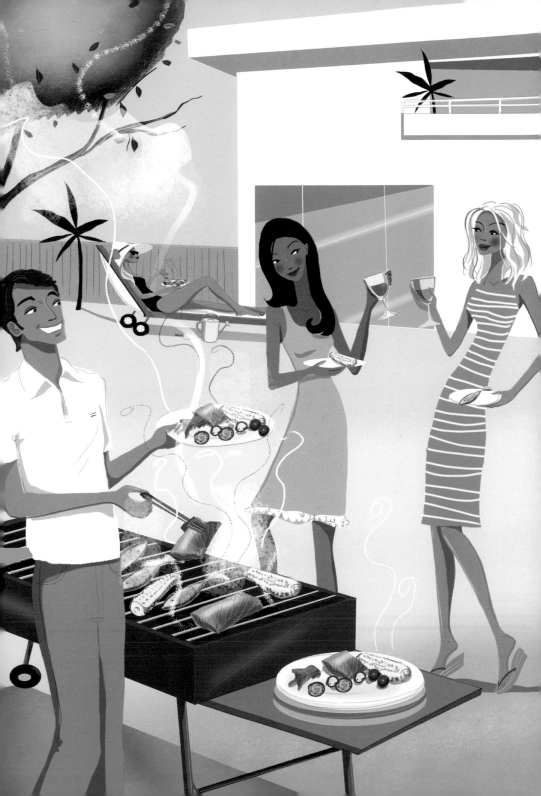

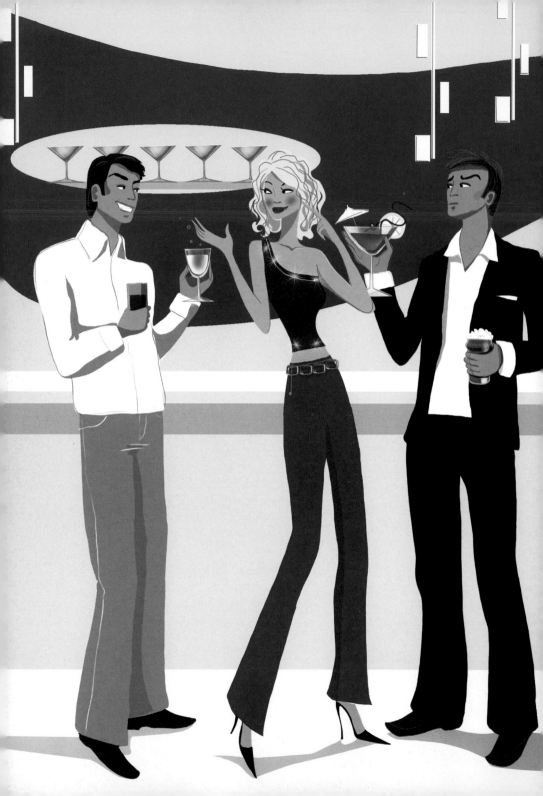

THE GOOD BOOZE GUIDE

Sadly, there's no getting away from the fact that all alcohol is high in calorific content. However, this doesn't necessarily mean an end to cocktails with friends and a bottle of wine with dinner. When it comes to **diet-friendly** booze, there's the good, the bad and the downright ugly. As a rule, when you're out for the night, the best drinks to stick to are dry white wine or **clear spirits**, with a low-calorie mixer such as a diet tonic or a cola drink. Drinks that health-conscious girls need to watch out for include: sugary alco-pops and cream-based **cocktails** such as Piña Coladas and White Russians.

★**TIP** Don't order bar snacks.
They're usually packed with hidden
calories and salt, which makes you
drink even more.

KNOW THE CALORIES YOU'RE DRINKING
PER STANDARD MEASURE

Best of a bad bunch
Vodka and diet cola
Dry white wine
Red wine
Champagne
Bottle of beer
Strawberry daiquiri
Bloody Mary
Manhattan
Baileys

The slippery slope down
Rum and cola
Gin and tonic
Margarita
Screwdriver
Tequila Sunrise
Bacardi Breezer
Singapore Sling
Piña Colada
White Russian

EAT TO **BEAT WRINKLES**

It's not only what you put on your skin that can help prevent wrinkles but also what you put into your body. No amount of expensive lotions and potions will stave off the ravages of time unless you're eating the right anti-ageing foods. This means eating more antioxidants – foods that are rich in nature's defence chemicals.

Antioxidants are important because they fight off free radicals – harmful molecules that are produced as a by-product of normal bodily functions and also stem from exposure to external toxins such as cigarette smoke, UV light and pollution. Free radicals **attack the cells** in our body and speed up the ageing process. Antioxidants are the body's **secret weapon** in fighting back, which is why filling our bodies with antioxidants from the food we eat can help keep us looking young.

Studies have been conducted to find out which foods contain the most antioxidants, notably reports from Tufts University in Boston. The result was a scoring system known as the ORAC score – the more **antioxidants** a food contains, the higher its score. Brightly coloured fruit and vegetables tend to have the best ORAC scores.

★TIP One trick to getting the right mixture of antioxidants is to think of making a fruit and vegetable rainbow as you shop for ingredients – try to include as many different colours as possible.

TOP TEN ANTI-AGEING FOODS

According to scientists, in order to get the maximum anti-ageing protection possible, you should aim to munch your way through between 3,000 and 5,000 ORAC units per day. Try to include as many of the foods below in your diet as possible. Scores are for 100 g (3½ oz) quantities.

1 **Prunes** ORAC score 5,770

2 **Raisins** ORAC score 2,830

3 **Blueberries** ORAC score 2,400

4 **Strawberries** ORAC score 1,540

5 **Spinach** ORAC score 1,260

6 **Brussels sprouts** ORAC score 980

7 **Broccoli** ORAC score 890

8 **Beetroot** ORAC score 840

9 **Avocado** ORAC score 782

10 **Oranges** ORAC score 750

Meal makeovers: how to age-proof your daily diet

Breakfast

Before A bowl of cornflakes with full-fat (whole) milk and a mug of coffee or tea.

After A bowl of porridge (oatmeal) made with soya milk, a handful of blueberries and prunes, plus a glass of fresh orange juice.

Lunch

Before A ham and cheese sandwich on white bread, plus a bar of chocolate.

After Low-fat cottage cheese with red pepper, baby spinach leaves and tomatoes on wholegrain bread and a fruit yogurt.

Dinner

Before White pasta with carbonara sauce, a glass of white wine and a chocolate mousse.

After Wholemeal (wholewheat) pasta with tomato sauce cooked with chilli, garlic and broccoli, a glass of red wine and a fresh fruit salad containing oranges, strawberries and kiwi.

WHAT TO EAT AND WHEN

Whether you're stressed, tired or in need of energy in order to hit the gym, what you choose to eat can make all the difference to how you feel and perform. Although it's easy to reach for the immediate fix that high-fat, sugar-laden foods give, the comfort will be short-lived and you'll feel worse for it in the long run. Read on to discover what to eat to help you cope.

YOU'RE FEELING STRESSED

Calm down with comfort foods that are rich in starch and B vitamins, which help the nervous system function properly. Good choices include wholegrain cereals, rice, potatoes and low-fat dairy products.

Try A bowl of porridge (oatmeal) topped with a sliced banana **or** a boiled egg with wholemeal (wholewheat) toast.

THE AFTERNOON ENERGY DIP

Choose food that is rich in protein to help you feel more energized. It will give you longer-lasting stamina than a bar of chocolate or cola drink, which only supply a short energy burst, followed by a sharp slump.

Try A low-fat yogurt **or** a handful of unsalted peanuts.

YOU HAVE A **BIG DAY** AHEAD

Research by Kellogg's has shown that children who eat cereal for breakfast concentrate better at school. So take a tip from the kids and have a large bowl of cereal in the morning for slow-release energy. Just before you leave the house, have something containing a little caffeine for an extra kick.

Try a bowl of muesli with semi-skimmed (2 per cent) milk **or** a small cup of coffee with your usual breakfast.

Coffee facts

★ Reports in the *Journal of the American Medical Association*, which followed almost 15,000 Finnish people – renowned as the world's biggest coffee drinkers – found women who drank ten or more cups a day had a 79 per cent reduced risk of developing diabetes. Those who drank three or four cups daily had a risk reduction of 29 per cent.

★ Drinking coffee on a regular basis could help boost your brain power, especially if you're a woman, says a report from the *American Journal of Epidemiology*.

★ A study, published in the journal *Chest*, found that those who drank three cups of coffee a day were 28 per cent less likely to have an asthma attack than non-coffee drinkers.

YOU'RE ABOUT TO **EXERCISE**

Don't eat a big meal for at least two hours before strenuous exercise, as it will make you feel sluggish and tired. Avoid anything very sugary because too much sugar can actually lower your energy levels. Instead, choose slow energy-release foods such as wholemeal (wholewheat) pasta or low-fat protein like fish or beans.

Try A pasta salad made with tuna, peppers and beans **or** an apple and a handful of almonds.

AFTER YOU'VE EXERCISED

If you've been swimming, gone for a run or completed any other strenuous form of exercise, you'll need to replace the lost fluids and minerals. Soups and fruit juices are perfect for this, but so are potatoes, which have a very high water content that helps you rehydrate.

Try a potato-based soup with wholegrain bread **or** a glass of fresh apple or orange juice.

★**TIP** The best time to drink sports, or 'isotonic', drinks is after exercise, as they help your body top up on glycogen – the fuel that powers muscles and provides energy.

KEEPING YOUR DIET ON TRACK

Now the bad news: wonder diets may offer a quick fix, but they don't work long-term. Yes, you might lose weight initially but they're often hard to stick to, expensive and, more importantly, can be dangerous. The fact is, diets that are very low calorie or exclude major food groups are unlikely to provide all the **nutrients** your body needs. So, even if you lose a few pounds, your general health could suffer. You're more likely to achieve lasting results by following a **sensible plan**. And if your life is already pretty hectic, you'll actually find it easier learning basic, good nutrition habits rather than trying to stick to complicated, time-consuming rules that faddy diets often entail. Try the following tips to boost your diet motivation.

PHONE A **FRIEND**

When it comes to dieting, it's often easier to stick to a programme when you have **company**. So don't go it alone – enlist a friend to join you in your quest to lose weight. According to a study on lone dieters conducted by Western Human Nutrition Center in the USA, lone dieters lose less weight and are more stressed than those dieting in a group. Women have much greater **success** with diets if a partner or close friend does it with them. You can plan to celebrate your successes together by spending a day at the shops or going to the cinema and be there to offer each other support when the going gets tough.

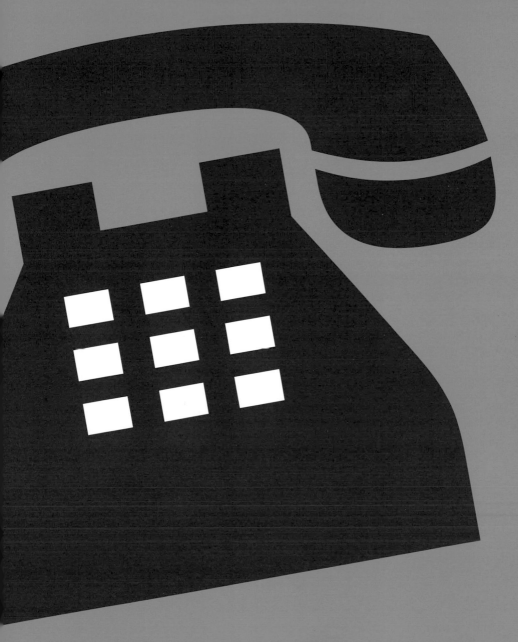

★**TIP** Make sure your phone-a-friend is someone with a positive attitude who doesn't give up easily – and not a pal who'll encourage you to share that chocolate eclair.

LEARN PORTION **CONTROL**

At each meal, aim to fill about half your plate with vegetables, one quarter with potatoes, pasta or rice and the final quarter with lean meat or fish. When you're eating out, always **resist the temptation** to super-size.

KEEP **MOTIVATED**

After the first few weeks of a diet boredom often sets in but don't give up; the trick is to stay motivated. Ring a good friend who has a positive 'can do' outlook on life and get them to give you a pep talk. This should help keep you focused on your goal of **getting in shape**. Also, try digging out some clothes catalogues or go bikini shopping – imagining how fantastic you'll look in that two-piece, after you've lost a stone, will soon get you back on track.

CHANGE YOUR HABITS

Make a permanent swap to healthy cooking methods. The best techniques are those that require little or no fat, so bake, steam or grill (broil) your food instead of frying, sautéing or roasting.

EAT ONLY WHEN YOU'RE **HUNGRY**

The best way to slim down and maintain your weight is to learn to eat only when you're hungry. Many of us eat as a result of stress, habit or boredom. When you feel the **urge to eat**, ask yourself whether it's true hunger you're feeling. Listen to your body's needs, even if this means eating six small meals rather then three main ones a day.

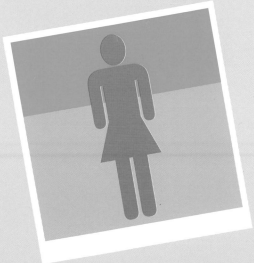

WATCH YOUR **ALCOHOL** INTAKE

It's amazing the amount of people who don't reduce the alcohol they drink when dieting, yet it's a sure-fire way to bump up those calories. You don't have to abstain, just **moderate your intake**. See page 137 to find out which drinks are the worst offenders.

HALT **HUNGER PANGS**

Drink plenty of calorie-free fluids such as water and herbal teas. We often mistake thirst for hunger, so try having a drink first and see if you still feel hungry after that. Similarly, don't confuse **hunger** with **appetite**. Real hunger is when your stomach is empty and your blood sugar is low, while appetite is the craving you get when you've had enough to eat but you can still smell something tasty like warm muffins or fresh bread.

KEEP A **REMINDER**

Find a photograph of how you looked before you started dieting and exercising and stick it on your fridge. Seeing how well you've done so far should give you the **incentive** to keep at it.

FIVE DIET CHEATS

Still finding it hard to stick to your diet? Try some of these effort-free tricks to help you eat more healthily.

GO FOR QUALITY NOT QUANTITY

Try putting less food on your plate. It may sound obvious but evidence from the University of Illinois in 2003 has shown that if food is in front of us we'll continue eating it, even when we're full. By the same token, we all tend to cook more food than necessary when preparing a meal. **Measuring** your amounts carefully will mean there are no 'seconds' to go back for!

CHOOSE FOODS THAT BOOST YOUR MOOD

What we eat can affect our emotions. Foods such as chocolate and cola drinks can have a negative effect on your mood because they give you a short **energy burst**, followed by a slump and they may induce feelings of guilt. Some **healthier** foods can actually stimulate the 'feel good' chemicals in the brain and make you feel happier and more relaxed. Good choices are oats, garlic, chilli, brazil nuts and bananas. The top four food 'stressors' to cut back on are: sugar, caffeine, alcohol and chocolate.

EAT **HEALTHY** COMFORT FOOD

Don't worry if you crave 'stodgier', more comforting foods in the winter. You can still follow a healthy diet by choosing fat-reduced versions of traditional favourites. For example, oven fries contain less fat than traditional fries. Try using olive oil to mash potatoes instead of butter and yogurt instead of cream with desserts. Remember that foods such as baked beans and porridge oats are all low fat but will leave you feeling full and **satisfied** when you eat them.

CHOOSE **SWEET NOT FATTY** FOODS

One of the main problems with chocolate, biscuits (cookies) and cakes is that they are high in fat as well as sugar. Because fat has twice the amount of calories as sugar, it's healthier to choose a treat that is sweet rather than fatty.

FILL UP WITH **SOUP**

Soup is the perfect meal. It is naturally low in fat, nutritious and very filling, especially if you choose to eat it with a chunk of wholegrain bread. Avoid soups that have cream added, as they contain more fat. Try to make your own fresh soup from scratch – **vegetable soup** or **gazpacho** is a great way to get three or four portions of vegetables.

THINKING THIN

You know the type. They seem to be able to eat whatever they feel like and never put on weight. Although the words 'I need to go on a diet' have never passed their lips, don't despise them completely. It's all to do with **mental attitude**! Read on to discover how you can learn some of the secrets of naturally skinny women.

A LITTLE OF WHAT YOU LIKE

When you're trying to lose weight, success is more likely if your diet is balanced and varied. Don't ban your favourite treats, like **sweets and cakes**, but include them in moderation. Denying yourself a particular food may lead you to binge on it later. Naturally skinny people tend to enjoy small **treats** when they feel like it, without gorging on them.

GET A GREAT START TO THE DAY

Skipping breakfast never helps you lose weight. According to a study by Professor Kirk, senior lecturer in nutrition at Queen Margaret University in Edinburgh, Scotland, eating breakfast can actually help you to **stay slim**. He found that people who ate a large bowl of cereal with semi-skimmed (2 per cent) milk every morning for 12 weeks lost around 1.5 kg (3 lb) more than those who didn't.

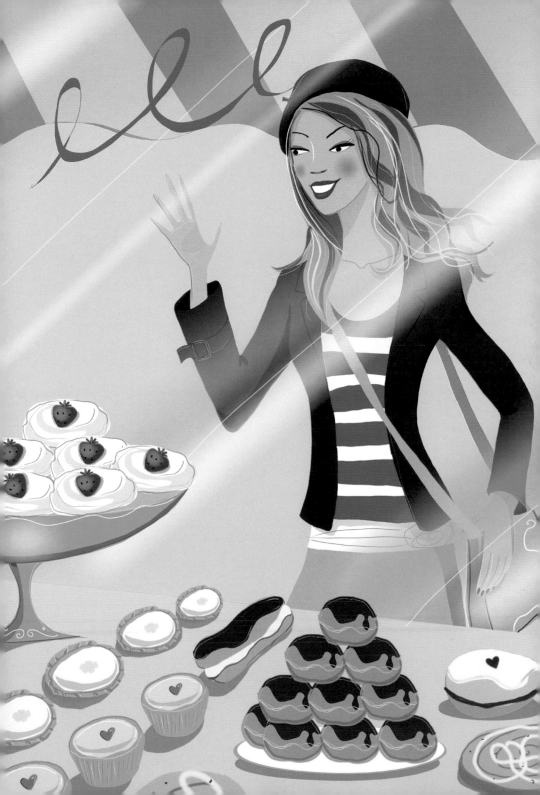

PICK FRUIT WISELY

When you first start a diet, try not to eat more than two portions of fruit a day, or you could notch up excess sugar and calories without realizing it. Apples, pears and berries are all good choices, but bananas are not (they have a high Glycaemic Index which can cause a **dip in energy** and mood). And be careful not to overdo the fruit juice.

SAVOUR YOUR FOOD

No one knows for sure how long it takes for your stomach to tell your brain that it's full, but dieticians estimate it is at least 10 minutes. So, do yourself a favour and slow down when you eat. **Pause** between each mouthful and chew everything properly. Put your knife and fork down between mouthfuls, pause between courses and take time to taste every bite. You'll be amazed at how **delicious** some of the food you usually take for granted actually tastes when you give yourself time to enjoy it.

THINK ABOUT WHAT YOU EAT

Next time you're feeling hungry, don't just stuff down the first bar of chocolate that you find. Stop and ask yourself how the food you want to eat will make you feel half an hour or so after you've eaten it. Will it give you energy or will it make you feel bloated and **full of guilt**? Think of a healthy alternative and how different it would make you feel, and then decide.

CHANGE YOUR **FOCUS**

One of the most important factors is the ability to believe you can be a slim person – something that slim people take for granted. If you think of yourself as overweight, you'll find it difficult to lose weight and keep it off. We tend to live up to our **self-image** so make a decision to start thinking positively today.

UNDERSTAND YOUR HUNGER

Slim people eat based on how hungry they are, so when lunch or dinner time comes around, they don't just fill up their plate because the food is there in front of them. Without thinking about it, they **judge how hungry** they are before they start eating. Similarly, if they feel full during a meal, they stop eating.

★**TIP** Try this trick to help you get in tune with your body. The next time hunger pangs strike, imagine you have a scale in your mind from one to five. One means you're not hungry, five means you're starving. Check where you are on that scale before you put anything into your mouth and only have something to eat if you think you're at least at hunger stage four.

DIET FACT FILES

The mind-boggling array of diets available can make it near impossible to decide which one to follow. There is an endless supply of books, videos and foods – many of which are endorsed by **celebrities** – to wade through. And while, in the long run, it's definitely better switching to sensible, healthy eating habits than following **faddy** food plans, some people find a set diet can help kick-start their weight loss. But which do you choose? Read on to get the lowdown on seven of the most popular diets available today.

THE **ATKINS** DIET
What is it?

A high-protein diet that severely restricts **intake of carbohydrates**. Unlike most conventional diets, the original nutritional plan didn't cut fat intake, although revisions have since recommended reducing saturated fat.

What can you eat?

Protein-rich meat, fish, eggs, **cheese**, nuts, cream and mayonnaise.

What's **banned?**

For two weeks there's a daily limit of 20 g carbohydrates, which means no fruit, bread, grains or **starchy** veg like potatoes. After this, you can increase your allowance in a controlled way.

How does it **work?**

The founder, Dr Robert Atkins, believed that our bodies produce too much insulin, which results in excess calories being stored as fat when we eat carbohydrates. A diet that is very **high in protein** is supposed to make our bodies burn fat instead of carbohydrates for fuel, resulting in weight loss in the process. Protein is also an appetite suppressant that can stop you feeling hungry.

Verdict

The jury remains out on this one. Recent trials have suggested that people lose weight quickly on this diet and may even experience a drop in cholesterol, though initial side effects include constipation and bad breath. There are also concerns over possible long-term **dangers** of this diet, particularly the strain it may put on the kidneys and heart.

THE **SOUTH BEACH** DIET
What is it?

Developed by Dr Arthur Agatston in 1999, this diet proved a **big rival** to the popular Atkins Diet. Just like Atkins, it works on the idea that carbohydrates cause weight gain. However, it does not eliminate them in quite such a ruthless fashion.

What can you eat?

The South Beach Diet divides carbohydrates into 'good' and 'bad' and is not quite so restrictive as Atkins. You can eat as many **good carbs**, such as vegetables and whole grains, as you like.

What's banned?

'Bad' carbs, such as cakes, **cookies** and white bread, and 'bad' fats, such as the saturated fats found in red meat and full-fat dairy products.

How does it work?

It's divided into three stages designed to provide quick **weight loss** at the beginning, followed by a more steady loss until you reach your ideal weight.

Verdict

Overall this is a good diet. It keeps your heart healthy and helps to reduce 'bad' cholesterol levels. It also seems to have one of the lowest dropout rates for modern diets and encourages **sensible eating patterns** that can be maintained long-term.

THE ZONE DIET
What is it?
Created by Barry Sears, the Zone Diet aims to give people the perfect balance of carbohydrates and proteins in order to regulate **blood sugar levels** and control weight.

What can you eat?
The Zone Diet recommends you eat 12 'zone blocks' a day – a block is a **balanced mix** of carbohydrate, protein and fat. Each 'zone' (or mini meal), carefully weighed out, should contain plenty of low-fat proteins, fruit and vegetables.

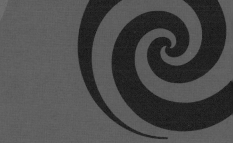

What's banned?
The diet advocates eating fewer carbohydrates such as potatoes, bread and pasta.

How does it work?
Sears believes eating in blocks encourages your body to burn off more fat, so you lose excess weight. Eating **little and often** rather than having three big meals keeps blood sugar levels constant, which avoids the energy crashes that can lead to bingeing. Plus eating small amounts regularly keeps your **metabolism** ticking over so you burn calories more efficiently.

Verdict
It's very low fat and contains plenty of health-friendly fruit and vegetables, but the lack of carbohydrates means it's not very high in fibre. Not an easy plan for busy girls to follow, as it is very **time-consuming** measuring out 12 mini meals a day.

FOOD COMBINING
What is it?

Dr William Hay invented Food Combining – also known as 'the Hay Diet' – in the early 1900s, not as a weight-loss diet but as a healthy eating plan. His theory centred on not mixing protein and carbohydrates at the same meal. He believed the two **food groups** 'fight' against each other in the stomach, causing digestive problems, weight gain and general bad health.

What can you eat?

As much fruit as you like throughout the day. At mealtimes you can either eat carbohydrates with vegetables or protein with vegetables.

What's banned?

Eating protein and carbohydrate at the same meal, plus white bread, rice and pasta, sugar and artificial additives.

How does it work?

Food combining doesn't promise weight loss, but is so **calorie-restricted** that you're bound to lose weight if you follow it properly.

Verdict

Although it's not bad for you nutritionally, this diet has very strict rules, making it difficult to follow, especially if your lifestyle is hectic – the **rules** mean never eating staples like cheese sandwiches or spaghetti with bolognaise sauce. Also, there is no actual scientific **evidence** to back the belief that the body can't digest protein and carbohydrates at the same time.

GLYCAEMIC INDEX (GI) DIET
What is it?

This diet is based on choosing carbohydrates that have low GI values. This means they break down into sugar very slowly and so have little effect on your blood sugar levels, leaving you **fuller for longer** and less likely to suffer from energy peaks and troughs.

What can you eat?

Any food with a low GI value, including apples, beans, oats and wholegrains.

What's banned?

All high GI foods such as **white bread**, white pasta, potatoes, dried fruits and bananas.

How does it work?

Because your blood sugar stays level, you don't get hungry and end up overeating, plus high GI foods tend to be **low in fat**.

Verdict

This is a sensible, low-calorie, low-fat diet that seems to work for many people. It contains plenty of fruit and vegetables and is very high in fibre, making it great for preventing heart disease and certain cancers. It's also good for keeping **energy levels** high.

MACROBIOTIC DIET

What is it?

A strict diet founded by George Ohsawa in Japan in the 1920s, which advocates eating organic, locally grown produce. The basic principle is to get a **perfect balance** of 'yin' and 'yang' foods to create overall good health.

What can you eat?

Around 50 per cent of the diet is based on **wholegrains**, such as brown rice, with the remainder made up from vegetables, beans and tofu.

What's banned?

It is essentially a vegan diet, so meat, eggs, **dairy**, alcohol, caffeine and any processed foods are off the menu.

How does it work?

Sweet foods are classified as 'yin' and savoury foods as 'yang'. Eating an equal balance of the two is supposed to create **harmony** in the body. It wasn't designed for weight loss, but the very low-calorie recipes will soon have most people shedding pounds.

Verdict

It is an extremely restricted diet and very time-consuming, as you have to really shop around to get the right organic ingredients and then spend hours preparing each meal from scratch. Plus, you may miss out on certain essential vitamins and minerals because you're **cutting out** whole food groups, including meat and dairy.

BLOOD GROUP DIET
What is it?

This diet is based on the idea that you should eat particular types of food according to your blood group. The creator, Peter D'Adamo, claims this will help you to lose weight, boost your energy and **strengthen** your immune system.

What can you eat?

Blood **group O**, for example, can eat as much meat as they want, but should cut out carbohydrates and dairy. **Group A**, on the other hand, can tuck into plenty of grains and fish, but must avoid red meat. **Group B** can enjoy a large range of foods and for them a very varied diet is important; however, they tend to have a natural tolerance for dairy products.

What's banned?

Any food that doesn't suit your specific blood group, according to D'Adamo's guidelines.

How does it work?

D'Adamo believes that your blood group reflects your body **chemistry** and how it breaks down food. Eating food that suits your blood group is therefore supposed to boost your metabolism so you burn more fat and calories.

Verdict

There's no scientific research to suggest that your ability to digest different foods is related to your blood group. Many people are blood group O and so are recommended to follow a low-carbohydrate, high-protein diet. If you do **lose weight** on this diet, it's probably because you're eating fewer calories.

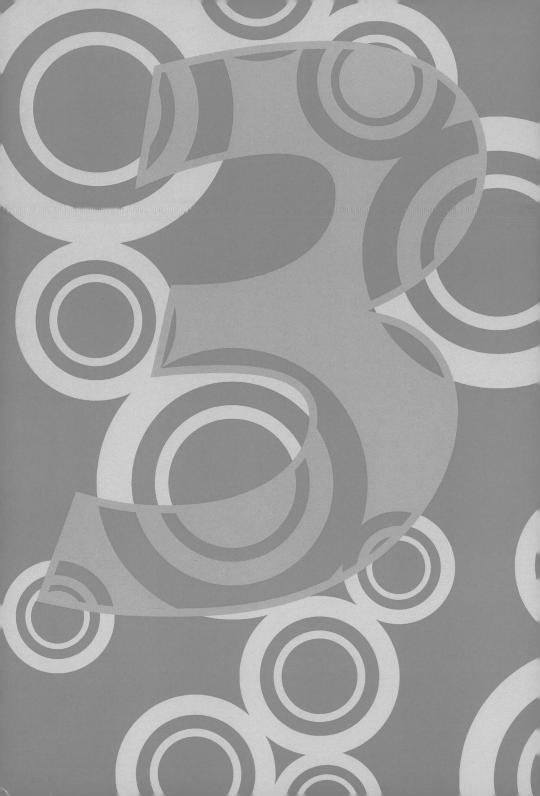

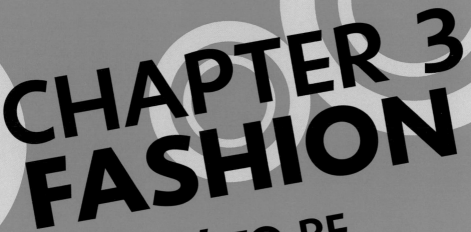

CHAPTER 3
FASHION

HOW TO BE
A STYLISH
BUSY GIRL

The ultimate step-by-step plan
to getting your wardrobe organized
and in shape fast, turning you into
the chic fashion icon you always
knew you were.

Every **busy girl** needs to know that there will always be something **stylish** in the wardrobe to wear – whether it's for work, a **hot date** or a walk in the park – and, what's more, must be able to find it **fast.** To do this, you need to build an affordable, capsule wardrobe with clothes to suit every **occasion**, plus become adept at a host of key style skills such as savvy shopping, learning how to translate catwalk to high street and picking the right shoes to create the perfect hemline-to-heel ratio.

You'll learn how to choose fabrics and cuts that flatter your figure, whatever your shape, and exactly how to strike that murky balance between underdressing and overdressing. With the help of this section, questions such as 'What belt should I wear to emphasize my waist?' and 'Which trousers will **hide my bum** while making my thighs look slimmer?' will become distant memories. And thanks to the style personality quiz, you'll finally be able to pinpoint 'your' look and make the most of it. At the same time, you'll discover what to pack to save precious minutes and space, whether you're off on a chic weekend **city break** or a sun-drenched beach holiday, as well as how to remedy any **fashion disaster** you may encounter as you go about your day.

CLEAR OUT YOUR CUPBOARDS

Like most truly busy girls, you've probably got a massive collection of clothes. Sadly, however, a bulging wardrobe and drawers so jam-packed they don't close don't automatically guarantee a host of chic, wearable outfits. Like everyone else, you probably have a surplus of tops that no longer fit, trousers that are too worn to wear and plenty of mistake buys that have never even made it out the front door. In order to streamline your clothes into a workable collection, you need to have a big clear out.

Pull everything you own out of the wardrobe and onto the bed, and take a critical look at what's there. Be ruthless! If it looks bad on you, you haven't worn it for two years or it's too big or too small, set it aside for charity. Do the same with your shoes. Anything with irreparable holes or splits should get thrown out. Now make a commitment to the **'two-year rule'** – if you haven't worn it in the last two years, you won't miss it and it's time it went.

Once you've finished, you will need to assess what's left and make a note of any significant gaps – for example, you might have loads of great tops, but a serious shortage of skirts and trousers. Don't hang onto 15 pairs of OK-fitting trousers; throw out all but the **most flattering** and make sure you have a range of different lengths to wear with heels and with flats. If you have short legs, get over-long trousers taken up so they look like they were made just for you.

> ### Have a clothes-swapping party
> Persuade some of your friends to clear out their wardrobes at the same time as you do, then throw a party. Get everyone together and have a great evening gossiping and swapping clothes. It's cheap, fun and sociable, and you get to breathe new life into each other's wardrobes.

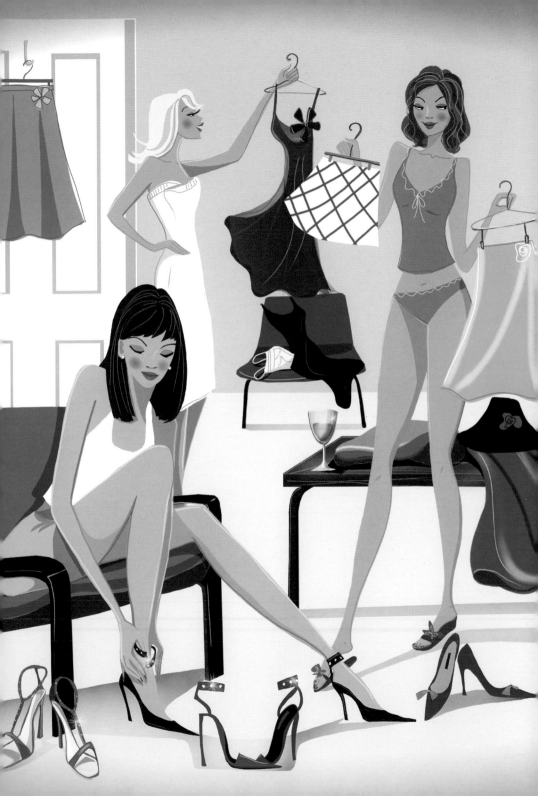

THE **RIGHT** FOUNDATIONS...

The key to an accessible, chic wardrobe is getting the basics right. To do this you need to compile a well-thought-out collection of clothes, with plenty of **fail-safe** outfits on hand. Once you have mastered this, all those 'I've got nothing to wear' days will become a thing of the past. Try not to think of a wardrobe full of **classics** as dull; the most effortlessly stylish people tend to wear timeless basics and use clever **accessories**, such as a brightly coloured top, a scarf or a trendy piece of jewellery, to **update** their look. So invest in some classic pieces that you can mix and match for any event and which will last for more than a season.

THE ITEMS YOU'LL **NEED**

One **good suit**

A classic trouser suit is worth spending time and money on. Do this and the suit should last you a good few years – the better the quality of the fabric and lining, the better the investment. A good suit can be the most **wearable and versatile** outfit you own, as it can be dressed up or down and worn separately with jeans or tops.

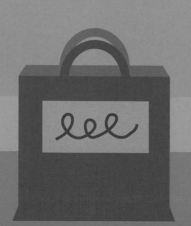

Coat

A good winter coat is one of the most important items you need to buy, so spend time getting the right one. You'll be wearing it most days when it's cold, so it needs to be versatile. Black is a **guaranteed safe colour** that never goes out of fashion and can be worn day or night. Go for a fine wool knit and keep the shape tailored but simple. Don't be tempted to go for the latest fur trim or funnel-neck shape – it will look dated by next year. Stick to a classic design and you will get years of wear out of it.

Length and cut is very important when choosing the **perfect fit**. A long coat worn with a short skirt is a cardinal fashion sin, so opt instead for long trousers and heels for a sleeker silhouette. Avoid mohair or angora scarves or sweaters if your coat is made of felt or wool – looking like you've been rolling around on the dog's blanket won't get you any style points!

Blazer

Make sure your wardrobe includes a good-fitting blazer, either in wool, corduroy or velvet. It is so versatile and you will be able to **team it** with everything from dresses to skirts and jeans for a smart-casual look.

Skirts

A dark, knee-length skirt is a fashion essential. A simple skirt can be worn with a plain, fitted top or shirt for the daytime and then vamped up with a **sexy, shimmery** top for the evening. Check out pages 194–8 for advice on which style of skirt best suits your body shape.

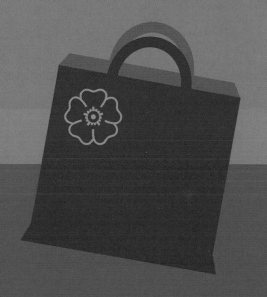

Dresses

A little black dress is a **party basic**. Choose one that is simple and well cut and can be worn in the day with a blazer or jazzed up with jewellery and glitzy shoes for the evening. See pages 213–14 for essential information on 'the little black dress'.

Trousers

Every wardrobe needs at least two pairs of smart, well-fitting trousers that can be worn with anything and make you feel great when you put them on. Tailored wide-cut or boot-cut shapes tend to **flatter everyone** and can be dressed up or down. It is also a good idea to have two pairs of well-fitting, classic jeans – one pair in a darker shade for winter and a second pair in a lighter colour for the summer months.

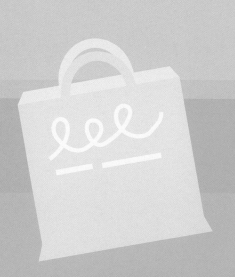

Tops

Fitted T-shirts and shirts in a wide variety of colours are the staple of any versatile wardrobe. For a great shape, choose fabrics with a hint of stretch but not too much or they tend to cling to your lumps and bumps. A classic **tailored shirt** will look great for work and can also be dressed down at weekends with jeans.

WHAT TO SPEND MONEY ON

'Buy the best of everything' is an outdated adage, never mind the financial implications, but certain items are still worth splurging out on – while with others you can get away with cheaper versions.

SPEND **WHAT YOU CAN** ON
- ✿ Coats
- ✿ Suits
- ✿ Shoes
- ✿ Handbags

SAFE TO **SAVE** ON
- ✿ Plain T-shirts
- ✿ Shirts
- ✿ Polo necks
- ✿ Summer dresses and skirts
- ✿ Scarves and belts

★**TIP** Finding it hard to budget for the clothes you want to buy? If you have to limit yourself to two items a month, then make one expensive but classic and the other cheaper but fun and of-the-moment. This way you can combine building the foundations of a great wardrobe with keeping up with the trends.

UNDERWEAR

It's easy to think you can get away with wearing shabby old underwear just because it's **hidden from sight**, especially if you are in a hurry to get ready in the morning. Badly fitting bras and pants, however, can ruin the shape and line of even the most expensive outfit, so invest in some smooth, well-shaped undies that fit you perfectly. They will streamline your curves and also help to improve your posture.

It is always worth getting your bra size measured professionally at your local department store or lingerie boutique – a recent UK survey found that 60 per cent of women were wearing the wrong size of bra. Make sure you have a good range of different bras to suit the varying necklines and backs of your clothes. A strapless, a halter neck and a backless bra should cover most dress shapes.

SIX SIGNS YOUR BRA IS NOT DOING ITS JOB

You can't wait to take your bra off the minute you walk through the door in the evening – it is probably the **wrong size**.

You look like you have four breasts. If your bra is too small, excess flesh will bulge over the top and ruin the line of your clothes – you need a **bigger size**.

Your bra rides up at the back – it is too big, which means your boobs are getting **no support**.

The underwire is popping out and into your flesh – **throw it away**!

It is cutting into your breastbone – it is **too small** or the straps are too tight.

You have **sore, red welts** on your shoulders by the end of the day – the bra is not supporting you enough.

Ten ways to ensure you always have something to wear

1 Stop impulse buying.
2 Clean out your closet.
3 Identify a wardrobe theme.
4 Pick two or three colours that will go with everything.
5 Work out what's missing from your wardrobe.
6 Only buy things that will work with something you already own.
7 Ignore the advice about buying the best of everything.
8 Buy more solid colour items than prints, as they are more versatile.
9 Try to add only two or three well-thought-out items to your wardrobe each month.
10 Continuously reassess your wardrobe and be ruthless. Get rid of any item that doesn't work, no matter how much you might like it.

THE INVISIBLE PANTY TRICK

Resolve your knicker dilemmas by having a different pair for every outfit scenario. These top five styles will help you look sleek and smooth without having to go commando.

✿ Flesh-coloured for white or see-through outfits.
✿ G-strings for clingy clothes that give you a VPL.
✿ Stretchy boy-style shorts for a smooth line under figure-hugging skirts.
✿ Hipsters for low-slung jeans and trousers.

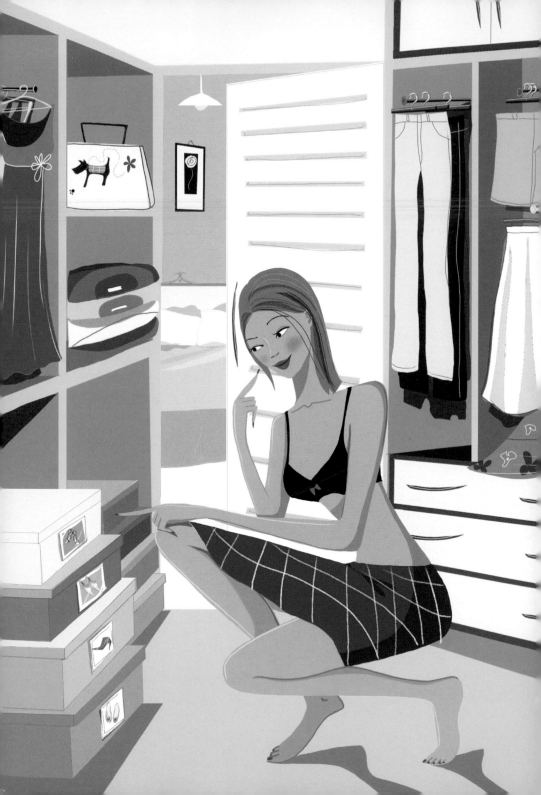

SPEEDY STORAGE SOLUTIONS

WARDROBE TOOLS

First, buy some good-quality wooden or padded coat hangers and chuck out all those freebie wire ones that can damage the shape of your clothes. **Group together** all your trousers, skirts, dresses and jackets so you know exactly where to look to find them. By being able to see what you have got, you will also start to wear all your clothes, instead of always choosing the things that are easiest to find. Store shoes in their boxes, to keep them protected, and write their colour, shape and size on the lid so that you know what's inside without having to open everything up. Ultra-organized girlies can **take a Polaroid** of each pair of shoes and stick it on the front of the box!

SHELVES

Fold up all your sweaters and chunky-knit cardigans and pile them on shelves according to colour and weight. This helps them keep their shape for longer and allows you to see what you have **at a glance** – put dark tones at the bottom and lighter colours on top. Freshly laundered winter sweaters can be put in plastic bags for storage during the summer months. T-shirts, scarves and jeans can be stored in this way too.

DRAWERS

Plastic drawer dividers are a great buy and will really help you get **organized**. Use them for separating your knickers, socks and tights for **fast access** in the mornings. Divide the sections into whites, colours and blacks; it is also worth separating black, navy and brown tights, so you don't pick the wrong colour on a dark morning. For **extra storage** space buy cardboard drawers to utilize the dead space at the bottom of your wardrobe – they are perfect for keeping belts, scarves and purses in order.

★**TIP** **Invest in some airtight plastic storage containers in which you can pack away off-season clothes. They will help prevent your clothes gathering dust or being attacked by moths when not in use.**

Daily **duties**

Resolve to make jumbled clothing a thing of the past. From now on every night you need to:

1 Put clean clothes away the minute you switch outfits.
2 Put dirty clothes in the laundry basket – invest in one that separates lights and darks for ease of laundering.
3 Fold and put away anything that can be worn again and hang up jackets, trousers and cardigans so you won't have to iron them again.

CARING FOR YOUR CLOTHES

It is all very well buying lots of gorgeous clothes, but unless you take good care of them, they won't last longer than a season. Hanging them up as soon as you take them off, washing them at the right temperature and removing stains as soon as they happen, will all ensure your clothes have a long and happy life and, more importantly, save you bags of time when you are getting ready in the morning.

COTTON

The most common natural clothing fibre is cotton. It is cool and **comfortable** and can be worn in both summer and winter, but it will shrink at high temperatures, so make sure you wash it at a maximum of 50°C (120°F). On the positive side, cotton irons well, especially while it is still damp; the negative side is that it needs ironing at all. Polyester and **cotton mixes** tend to be a bit more crease-resistant and are therefore less time-consuming as they don't need so much ironing, which makes them a good alternative.

★**TIP** Always check the labels on items before you wash them, but bear in mind that manufacturers often state 'dry-clean only' on clothing to cover themselves against liability if they become damaged in the wash. Woollen coats and suits should be dry-cleaned, but such fabrics as silk and cashmere can be gently hand-washed in cool water.

LINEN

One of the most durable natural fibres, linen is three times as strong as cotton. It is very **popular** for trousers and shirts in the summer as the fabric allows the skin to breathe and keeps you cool. On the downside, linen is prone to badly creasing, even when it has just been ironed. Always follow the **care instructions** on the label, as some linen must be hand-washed while other items can be machine-washed at a cool temperature.

WOOL

A very versatile fibre, wool can be either warm or cool depending on the type. Cashmere, one of the most expensive types of wool, is one of the softest and most **lightweight yarns** and can be worn whatever the weather. Cashmere and other similar delicate knits should always be hand-washed or dry-cleaned. Some other wool can now be washed in the machine, on a delicate wash, but always check the label and never wash at a high temperature, as all wool will shrink. When drying wool, never use the tumble dryer. Instead, let your garments dry naturally. As woollen clothes can lose their shape if hung to dry, the best thing to do is to roll the item in a towel, to **absorb excess water,** and then take it out and lie it flat to dry, keeping it away from direct heat.

SILK

Silk is one of the most luxurious fabrics but it can need specialist cleaning, so always check the label before washing. Some silks can be hand-washed in lukewarm water with a gentle detergent but others must be **dry-cleaned**. If you are washing silk by hand, make sure to add a few drop of gentle fabric conditioner to the final rinse to prevent static. Silk dries very quickly and should never be tumble-dried or placed near a direct heat source. Steam-iron **carefully** on a low heat by placing a cloth over the silk to protect it.

MANMADE FABRICS

Some manmade fabrics can be washed at higher temperatures, but you should always check the label first. Acrylics and nylons can melt at moderate to high temperatures, and other manmade fibres may deteriorate rapidly.

★**TIP** Rather than hand-washing delicate beaded or sequinned items, which means wringing out and possibly damaging them, place them in a tightly fastened pillowcase and wash them on the cold cycle in the washing machine.

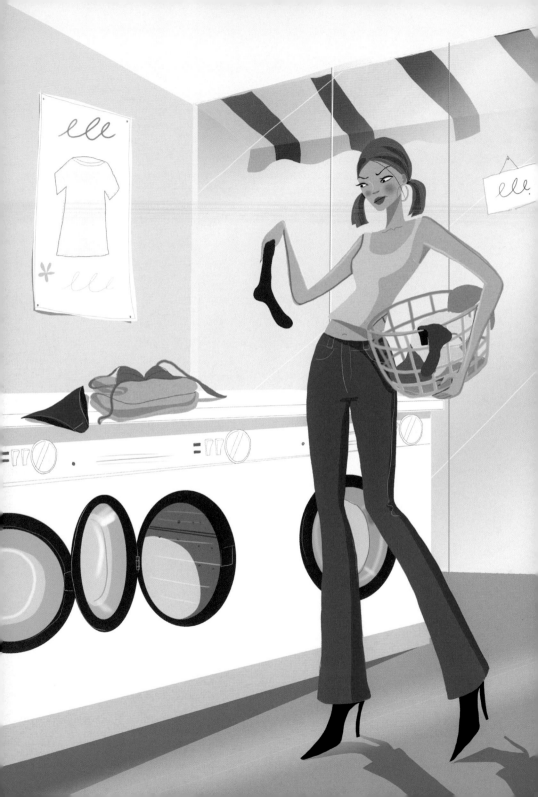

GETTING WASHING RIGHT

MACHINE WASHING

The first rule of machine washing is to make sure that you empty all the pockets – there is nothing worse than unloading a dark wash only to discover that everything is covered in white bits from the Kleenex you left in your jeans pocket. Also, turning jeans and denim jackets inside out will help to prevent them from fading. Follow your common sense and wash bright colours together, darks together and whites together. If something is covered in mud, wash it on its own and any clothes that shed fibres, such as towels and fleeces, should also be washed separately to avoid covering everything else in fluff. Always check the labels on all garments to make sure that you don't exceed the recommended maximum temperature and risk ruining items. Finally, make sure you don't **overload the machine** – too many items means they won't be washed as effectively and the strain of a heavy load may shorten the life of your washing machine. If you're in a major hurry and don't have time to wait for your machine to run through a full cycle, most machines have a quick wash button for loads in half the time.

★**TIP** Try adding fabric conditioner to your wash to make clothes easier to iron and save time.

HAND-WASHING

Using hot or warm water when hand-washing is a common mistake. To avoid damaging delicate fabrics, always use cold water and never leave things to soak or they might shrink! Add the recommended amount of hand detergent to the cold water and gently move the garment around in it, squeezing rather than rubbing. Rinse thoroughly in fresh cold water until it runs clear and carefully squeeze, **do not wring**, the water out or roll in a towel to remove excess moisture. Dry flat if the item is made of wool. To save drying time, some machines have a slow spin cycle that is great for getting moisture out of delicate clothes without damaging them.

DRYING

When you unload the machine, shake out the wet items to loosen creases; it will help to **save time ironing**. The tumble dryer can be a godsend when it comes to saving time and space but don't overload it and keep similar garments and fabrics together. Dry them for long enough to remove moisture and wrinkles but be careful; if you leave it on too long the heat can set the wrinkles, increase static and cause shrinkage. Hang your clothes up as soon as they come out of the washing machine or tumble-dryer to reduce ironing time. Clothes that can't be tumble-dried should be hung on hangers to dry naturally. Nondelicates will also dry very quickly on a medium-heat radiator.

IRONING

Possibly the dullest task known to man! Try to minimize the amount of ironing you do by hanging everything up straight away to dry and with a bit of luck it won't even need to be ironed. If you have to iron, make sure you read the **care label** for the correct temperature setting for the fabric you are ironing. Don't iron clothes that are stained as the heat may seal the stain in, making it harder to remove. Anything delicate should be ironed on the reverse side or under another cloth to protect the fabric.

SMELL **SWEET**

Scented waters, such as lavender water, are a great way to infuse a subtle smell into your clothing. Add scented water to an iron and, using it on steam setting, gently waft it over clothing. This is also a great way to **freshen clothes** that have been in storage.

★**TIP** By selecting your clothes the night before, you will save time and stress the following morning. It will also prevent those time-consuming clothes-flinging scenarios, where you try on everything you own only to settle on the first outfit you tried on!

Clothes **check**

1 To avoid last-minute panics in the morning, set aside one hour a week to iron, organize dry cleaning, and sew on buttons or tidy hems.

2 Make one evening a week 'wash night'. It may sound boring but you will avoid the situation where the top you want to wear is dirty. Make it more fun by playing music or chatting to a friend on your hands-free phone as you go.

3 Check out your local dry-cleaning delivery service. They make life easier by picking up and dropping off items at a time convenient for you.

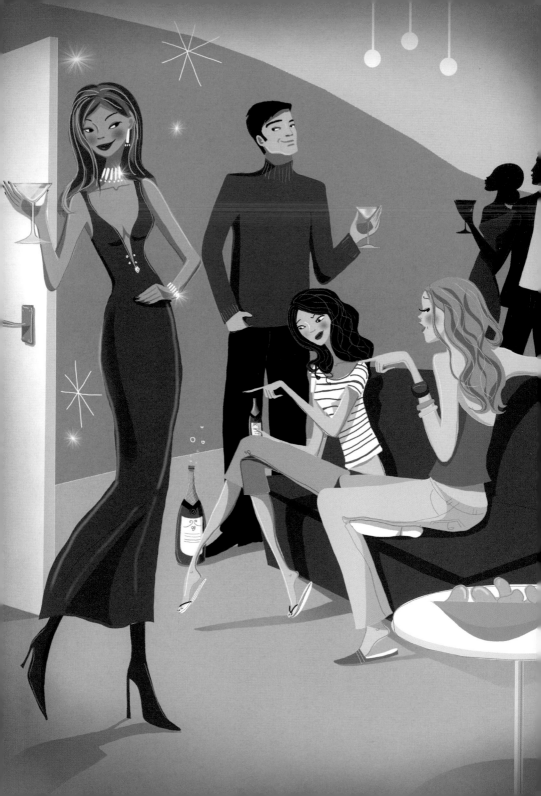

WHAT'S YOUR **STYLE PERSONALITY?**

Identifying the type of clothes you are most drawn to can help you create a signature look, which will save lots of time when shopping or getting ready to go out. If you are not sure about the type of look you want to achieve, try answering these questions:

Q1 WHAT IS YOUR FAVOURITE FASHION DECADE?
A 2030!
B 1890s.
C 1940s.
D Now.
E 1980s.

Q2 YOU ARRIVE AT A PARTY AND REALIZE YOU ARE TOTALLY OVERDRESSED. HOW DO YOU HANDLE THE SITUATION?
A I enjoy being in the spotlight and try to attract as many stares as possible.
B I don't really mind – I'm used to dressing in clothes that are a bit different.
C I take off my jacket and pop to the toilet to tone down my make-up and accessories.
D I leave the party as soon as possible.
E I feel a bit self-conscious but after a couple of drinks forget about it.

Q3 YOU ARE BEING TAKEN OUT FOR A MEAL. WHERE WOULD YOU PREFER TO GO?
A The latest place favoured by the fashionista.
B A small and romantic Italian.
C Your favourite restaurant, where you know the food will be fantastic.
D Somewhere you can enjoy a healthy meal, such as the local Japanese.
E Somewhere expensive where you can really dress up to the nines.

Q4 YOU ARE MEETING UP WITH THE GIRLS. HOW DO YOU DRESS?

A I'll wear the up-to-the-minute jacket and shoes I bought in a designer boutique last week.

B I'll wear my favourite beaded top with a pretty floral skirt.

C I'll wear something classic and understated, such as a white shirt, navy blazer and well-fitting jeans.

D I'll wear something comfortable – I don't need to show off in front of my friends.

E I'll wear a sexy outfit – you never know who you are going to meet...

Q5 WHAT KIND OF MUSIC DO YOU LISTEN TO?

A I listen to anything that's new on the radio. That way I know what's currently 'in'.

B Jazz or classical music is my favourite.

C I stick to the music of my favourite artists and buy all their CDs.

D Anything that's fast and upbeat.

E Something slow and sexy.

Q6 WHAT IS YOUR FAVOURITE ITEM OF CLOTHING?

A Cutting-edge jacket.

B Vintage blouse.

C Cashmere sweater.

D Comfy tracksuit.

E Sexy black dress.

Q7 WHAT IS YOUR FAVOURITE FABRIC?

A Denim.

B Lace.

C Cashmere.

D Fleece.

E Silk.

Q8 WHICH WORDS BEST DESCRIBE THE KIND OF CLOTHES YOU LOVE?

A Bold, creative and edgy.

B Feminine, soft and flowing.

C Tailored, understated and elegant.

D Easy, casual and comfortable.

E Chic, sexy and seductive.

MOSTLY 'A'S – THE TREND SETTER

It is important to you that you are always dressed in up-to-the-minute clothes and your trusty copy of *Vogue* is never far from your side. You love **experimenting** with make-up and changing your hairstyle and colour but once everybody else catches on and a particular fashion becomes widespread you stop wearing it immediately. You keep an **eye on the catwalks** and seek the unusual in fashion so you should make this the keynote of your style, drawing on ideas from different parts of the world to achieve your individual look.

How to avoid becoming a fashion victim

❀ Make sure you are not wasting too much money on fads by assessing the last five items you bought – if three or more could be classed as this season's 'must haves' you are in danger of turning into a fashion victim.

❀ Before buying, ask yourself how much you really love the item and if you will still be able to wear it next year.

❀ Never mix more than two different trends together.

❀ Remember, models and celebs often over-do looks for maximum photo impact, which probably won't translate well on a day-to-day basis for you.

MOSTLY 'B'S – **BOHO BELLE**

You love vintage clothes and jewellery and spend hours in charity shops and flea markets picking up unique, but beautifully made, pieces. You prefer loose, flowing and **sensual clothes**; for you, the feel and colour of the fabric is just as important as the shape. You don't follow fashion and aren't interested in the latest fads. You are very creative, but a bit of a dreamer.

How to avoid looking **stuck** in the **past**

✿ Try to incorporate some modern pieces into your existing wardrobe.

✿ Look for modern takes on classic clothes, such as blouses with Victorian-style puff sleeves.

✿ Look for high street imitations of vintage jewellery – it costs far less but still looks very authentic.

MOSTLY 'C'S – **CLASS ACT**

Your style is a study in balance and harmony, which shows the world that you possess a subtle knowledge about the art of dressing well. You are **up-to-date** on all the latest fashion looks but you don't follow them slavishly, which sets you apart from the others. Style to you is captured in the fine details of a garment and how it is created. Your style suggests **simplicity and elegance** combined with timelessness and perfectly reflects your great sense of occasion. Having immaculately groomed hair and make-up is very important to you.

How to **stop** your **wardrobe** becoming dull

✿ Classy girls often stick to neutrals, which is fine for most of your wardrobe but colour is important for adding glamour and punch, if you know how to use it.

✿ Choose a few key items, such as tops and accessories, to inject some colour into your look.

✿ Don't stray too far from your normal style, as you have a natural instinct for what suits you.

MOSTLY 'D'S – **SPORTY BABE**

You love the outdoors and spend a lot of time exercising. Style is not top of your list, although you do like to choose **good-quality** sportswear to show off the toned body you've worked so hard to achieve. You favour clothes with a no-nonsense style that allow you freedom of movement. You like to keep hair and make-up simple and easy to maintain.

How to **look sporty** without losing **smart**

- ✿ Always keep clothes pressed and in good condition.
- ✿ Wear layered coordinates and pull them together with a blazer.
- ✿ Headwear, such as baseball caps, can give many smart-casual outfits a laid-back sporty look.

MOSTLY 'E'S – **SEXY SIREN**

Clothes are a way of expressing your sexuality and conveying your magnetic personality. Glamour is all-important and you spend hours getting ready – even for a quiet drink. You are never seen without your make-up and you like clothes that show off your body – you aren't afraid to wear short skirts or low-cut dresses. **Killer heels** are a staple and you own a vast shoe collection.

How to avoid **over-vamping** it

- ✿ Wear flesh-coloured underwear with white clothes or anything remotely see-through – underwear on show is never sexy.
- ✿ If you have big boobs, don't wear long pendants that nestle in your cleavage – it looks tacky.
- ✿ Show off your boobs, your legs or your bum, but never more than one.

★**TIP** Whatever your style personality, avoid wasting time and money by referring back to the three words you choose in the quiz to sum up the kind of clothes you love. If you ticked 'feminine, soft and flowing', be honest and question if the item fits that description. Although not everything you buy has to be in exactly the same style, it will give you a more objective viewpoint when asking yourself, 'Is this really me?'

BE YOUR OWN
PERSONAL SHOPPER

Now you've cleared your wardrobe and have a better idea of your **individual style personality**, it's time to hit the shops! Here we look at how to fill in the gaps in your clothing collection, while avoiding those impulse buys.

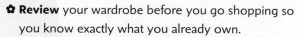

GETTING **THE MOST** FROM YOUR **SHOPPING TRIP**

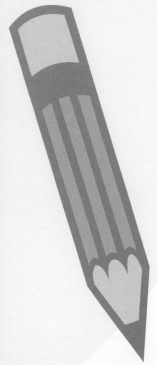

- ✿ **Review** your wardrobe before you go shopping so you know exactly what you already own.
- ✿ Save **tear sheets**. Every time you see a top or skirt you like in a magazine, rip it out and keep them in your handbag for instant inspiration.
- ✿ Make a **list** of exactly what you need – be it a coat, a pair of black boots or a top to go with that skirt you've never found a match for.
- ✿ **Fix your price**. You need to set a budget, be firm with yourself and don't go over it. If you know you can't control yourself, get your day's budget from the cash machine and leave credit and store cards at home.
- ✿ **Prioritize**. What is the most important purchase you want to make? If you won't feel satisfied unless you go home with the perfect coat, don't allow yourself to be distracted by other items until you've found it.
- ✿ **Take it with you**. If you have a favourite skirt but have never found anything to wear with it or a top that none of your bottoms quite match, take it with you – make it your mission to **find its perfect partner**!
- ✿ Make a list of '**must visit**' shops. Knowing exactly where you want to go will stop you wasting time and energy in 'so-so' shops.

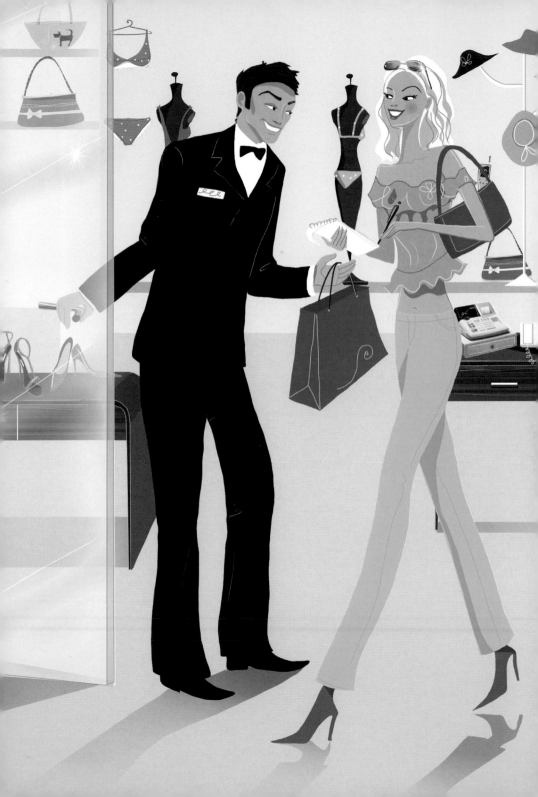

- ✿ Get your outfit **right**. Wear clothes that are easy to take on and off, without making you look like a rumpled mess. Wear streamlined but supportive **underwear**, so that you won't spoil the look of any clothes you try on, and do your hair and make-up so you see yourself in the best light.
- ✿ Go it alone or with one good mate. If you really need a **second opinion**, you can always try it on at home and ask someone then. Always check the shop accepts returns first, though.
- ✿ Give yourself **plenty of time**. Shopping when you are in a hurry or thinking about other things is a bad idea. You will end up rushing and buying something in haste that you will probably hate when you get home. If you are going shopping with a friend after a big lunch, stick to mineral water – many a disastrous fashion choice has been made after a glass or two of Chardonnay!
- ✿ Don't shop when you are feeling down. You will end up buying **mistake items** or being over-critical of yourself, which will make you feel worse. Go to see a film or meet a friend for lunch for a more effective pick-me-up.
- ✿ Ask yourself these three questions before you buy anything. **Does it fit?** Does it go with what I already have? Does it suit me?
- ✿ Check the **washing instructions** – does it still seem so gorgeous if you have to hand-wash or dry-clean it after every wear?
- ✿ If you find a pair of trousers or a skirt that is the perfect fit, consider buying more than one pair, especially if they are black. Black tends to fade after a while, but with **two pairs** of the same trousers the wear and tear will take longer.
- ✿ Beware of **misleading 'skinny' mirrors** in department stores and boutiques. If a style didn't look good on you in the past, it won't now – unless you've made some major changes to your diet and exercise regime.

SPEEDY SALES SHOPPING

HOW TO BUY CLOTHES TWICE AS STYLISH IN HALF THE TIME

It's a myth that you have to spend hours trawling through the shops to get the best buys at the sales. Here's how to hunt down a real bargain and avoid wasting time and money on items you don't ultimately want.

Decide what you are looking for and stick to it – it's only a bargain if you needed it in the first place.

Only buy things in the right size and that **fit perfectly** – the exceptions to this rule are trousers or skirts that simply need taking up in length.

Think comfort. Anything that feels uncomfortable when you first try it on will be murder by the end of the day!

Stick to classics. That orange and blue miniskirt might be very this season, but how will it look **next year**? You are better off sticking to simple, timeless pieces.

If you can't see yourself wearing it on at least **three different occasions** (unless it is sportswear or a wedding dress of course!) don't buy it.

Don't buy anything in a sale that you would not pay **full price** for.

Colour coordination

Have you ever taken a moment to stop and think about which colours actually suit you? Just because turquoise is your favourite colour, that doesn't mean it will look good when you wear it. A quick and easy way to work out your 'colours' is to grab a selection of different-coloured tops in a shop and try them on one after another. The ones that give your face and skin an instant lift are the colours you should be choosing to base your wardrobe around.

DRESSING TO SUIT YOUR SHAPE

When it comes to getting ready in a hurry, you don't want to waste time hunting for a decent outfit in your wardrobe. It makes sense to follow a few guidelines on dressing for your body shape. Stick to these basic rules and you'll avoid spending hours trying everything on in the morning as you'll be safe in the knowledge that all your clothes have been bought to suit your shape and flatter you. There are four main body types, so pick the one that best describes you and read on to discover what you should be wearing:

APPLE
MAIN CHARACTERISTICS
- You tend to carry fat around your stomach.
- You have a full waist, upper back and bust.
- Your bottom is small and flat.
- Your shoulders seem wider than your hips.
- Your waist is a similar width to your hips.
- Your thighs tend to be lean and rarely carry excess weight.

BEST CLOTHES CHOICES FOR YOUR SHAPE
- Try loose, unstructured jackets over slim-fitting dresses.
- Make your top-heavy figure look longer and slimmer by wearing all one colour.
- Accentuate narrow hips with sexy pencil skirts.
- Choose well-cut trousers with straight legs to emphasize your legs' slim shape.
- Wear short skirts with bare legs or flesh-coloured tights to draw attention to your shapely legs.

AVOID
- Fitted shirts or jackets – they will only draw attention to your bulky top half.
- Heavy-knit sweaters or cardigans, for the same reason.

PEAR

MAIN **CHARACTERISTICS**

- ✿ You tend to carry fat on your bottom and hips.
- ✿ You have a well-defined waist and large, curvy bottom.
- ✿ Your hips are wider than your shoulders.
- ✿ Your bust is quite small.
- ✿ Your stomach is flabby.
- ✿ Your thighs are prone to heaviness.

BEST CLOTHES **CHOICES** FOR YOUR SHAPE

- ✿ Try belts that can be drawn in to accentuate your waist but don't pull them in too tight or your hips will be highlighted.
- ✿ Wear patterns on your top half to draw attention away from your lower half.
- ✿ Choose boot-cut trousers over straight leg to balance out your big thighs.
- ✿ Go for tailored jackets and shirts that cover your bottom.
- ✿ Choose eye-catching jewellery and scarves to take the attention away from your hips.

AVOID

- ✿ Skin-tight trousers and pencil skirts as they make your thighs look bigger.
- ✿ Very short skirts and dresses, as they will make your hips look wider and your legs shorter.
- ✿ Any clothes that are too tight – choosing the next size up will make you look slimmer and no one will ever know what size you are wearing.

HOURGLASS

MAIN CHARACTERISTICS

✿ You tend to carry fat equally over your whole body.
✿ Your hips and shoulders are a similar width.
✿ You are very curvy.
✿ Your waist is narrow and well toned.
✿ Your stomach is flat and toned.
✿ Your thighs can look heavy.

BEST CLOTHES CHOICES FOR YOUR SHAPE

✿ Make the most of your sexy shape with close-fitting dresses.
✿ Choose clothes that accentuate the narrowness of your waist.
✿ Opt for thin belts rather than wider ones to define your waist even more.
✿ Invest in good-quality underwear to give your bust and bottom support and shape.
✿ Try 1940s-style tea dresses and 1950s glamour gowns to make the most of your shape.

AVOID

✿ Very short skirts as they will make your bottom look bigger.
✿ Baggy, untailored clothes that will hide your curves and make you look heavier than you are.

ATHLETIC

MAIN **CHARACTERISTICS**

✿ Your bust and hips are a similar width.

✿ Your bust is fairly small.

✿ You have no real waist.

✿ Your figure is pretty much straight up and down.

✿ Your bottom is small and flat.

✿ Your legs are long and slim.

BEST CLOTHES **CHOICES** FOR YOUR SHAPE

✿ Add definition to your waist with an eye-catching belt, either thick or thin.

✿ Wear one solid colour from top-to-bottom for elegance.

✿ Find ornate necklaces and earrings to draw attention to your slender neck and shoulders.

✿ Choose soft, flowing fabrics that soften your shape to add femininity.

✿ Go for shapes that accentuate your waist, such as drawstring trousers or belted dresses.

AVOID

✿ Anything with square or big shoulders – it will draw attention to your lack of shape.

✿ Very tailored suits that can make you look shapeless.

✿ Wide-legged trousers – they will simply emphasize your lack of curves.

SLIM WEAR

No one is 100 per cent happy with their body so, when time is of the essence and you need to look – and feel – ten pounds thinner, try some of the following optical illusion, spot-reducing tricks.

FOR A FULL BUST

A sleeveless turtleneck **diverts attention away** from a busty upper body by emphasizing the arms. Similarly, a cropped jacket will draw the eye to the waist. Always wear a good supportive bra that will lift your boobs.

FOR HEAVY LEGS

Boot-cut trousers and skirts with a **small side split** work well. Wear trousers and skirts that are on the large side rather than too tight – anything that appears to be straining at the seams will only make you look bigger.

FOR BIG HIPS

Choose **A-line skirts** and plain colours. You should also avoid shiny, satin fabrics or bright-coloured skirts and trousers, which will draw attention to saddlebags.

FOR THICK ANKLES

Don't wear strappy delicate heels as they will draw attention to the ankle area. Also avoid **flat ballet pumps** or shoes with ankle straps that cut across the ankles and make them look bigger.

FOR A BIG BOTTOM

A long-line blazer will hide your behind and give you the confidence to wear a **body-fitting dress** or straight-leg jeans. Avoid G-strings, as they can accentuate a large backside, and instead choose hipster briefs, with plenty of Lycra support, to lift your bum and prevent it looking saggy.

How to choose the **best bikini**

Sunbathing on the beach is about as close as most of us get to taking all our clothes off in public, so it's no wonder it can be a bit daunting! No matter how **healthy or fit** you are, some parts of your body are bound to cause concern. Follow the guide below to make sure you choose the right bikini for your shape.

★ **Short neck**
Choose plunging necklines but steer clear of halter necks as they will draw attention to the problem.

★ **Narrow shoulders**
Go for boob tube-style, bandeau tops that will help make your shoulders look broader.

★ **Broad shoulders**
Halter necks are the best style to draw attention away from wide shoulders.

★ **Big bust**
Choose something with plenty of support to prevent boobs from looking saggy.

★ **Flat chest**
Opt for cups that contain some padding to boost your bust.

★ **Short body**
Pick vertical stripes that will help make your body look longer.

★ **Pot belly**
Cover a big tummy with shorts-style bottoms or a swimsuit with added control.

★ **Wide hips**
Pick bikini tops with plenty of detail to draw the eye away from your bottom half.

★ **Chunky thighs**
Wear a sarong over your bikini or choose longer, shorts-style bottoms.

★ **Large bum**
Choose a light coloured bikini for a size-minimizing effect.

★ **Short legs**
Choose a high-cut, skimpy bikini to add length to your legs.

★**TIP** Always pack a sarong for beach breaks. It can be used to cover a multitude of sins and is the ultimate speedy outfit. Wrap it around your body and tie it behind the neck for a simple sundress in which you can hit the bar straight from the beach.

HOW TO USE CLOTHES
TO LOOK SLIMMER

DO Wear prints with dark backgrounds to create an overall illusion of slenderness.

DO Wear block colour from head-to-toe in a clean unbroken line – it can have a dramatically slimming effect.

DO Wear suits instead of dresses. The more lines and seams there are, the less attention will be paid to any bulges.

DO Wear empire-line dresses. They have high waists and will flare out and skim your body from your bust down. They are more forgiving for areas like the hips and tummy.

DON'T Wear pleats – they add pounds.

DON'T Wear brown and navy thinking they have the same slimming effect as black – they don't!

DON'T Wear Lycra or other stretchy fabrics – they are very unforgiving!

★**TIP** Be careful with prints, as they can create optical illusions. The main point to remember is that tiny prints will make a big girl look bigger and big prints will dwarf a tiny girl.

HOW TO USE CLOTHES
TO LOOK TALLER

DO Go for a solid-coloured, matching skirt or trouser suit to create a long, lean line.

DO Stick to dresses that are simple and classic, avoiding fussy details.

DO Wear the same tone of colour in shoes, tights, skirts and jackets. It will elongate the silhouette and make you look taller.

DON'T Wear shoes with heels that are too high or else they will look out of proportion.

DON'T Go for girlie details. Ruffles or bows will make you look shorter.

HOW TO USE CLOTHES
TO LOOK SHORTER

DO Choose double-breasted jackets. They are very flattering and help normalize extreme proportions.

DO Opt for large jewellery so everything looks in proportion.

DON'T Wear anything skimpy or too short. Jackets should fall below the hips.

DON'T Wear completely flat shoes. A small heel will create better balance.

DON'T Wear clothing that is too severe. Wearing a solid, dark, heavily constructed suit can appear quite masculine, so break up the line with softer, flowing fabrics in lighter shades.

WHAT TO WEAR

The key to good style is knowing what to wear and when. To do this successfully you need to make your wardrobe work for you. That means keeping it **flexible** and ensuring that you have something for **every occasion**. Appropriateness is the word here. However much you dress just for yourself at the weekend, when going for a job interview or to your best friend's wedding you need to stick to certain rules to look your best.

TO WORK

Wearing the right clothes to work can help your career progress, while inappropriate outfits may mean you are passed over for **promotion**. But these days it is not as simple as wearing a suit – what you wear depends on where you work. Here's how to dress to impress at the office.

YOUR FIRST JOB

When you go for your interview, check out what the other staff are wearing. Once you first start work it is important to be noticed for the **right reasons**: that is, your job skills and not your wacky dress sense. If appropriate wear a suit, or, for a less formal look, you can't beat a pair of well-cut trousers and a fitted top or shirt in a colour that suits your skin tone. Dress for the **job you want,** not the job you have. Even if you are only the office junior, presenting a well-groomed image may help you to fast-track your career.

IN THE **FINANCIAL DISTRICT**

Dark colours are more professional-looking than bright, so go for **chic** neutrals. A sexy, well-tailored suit is perfect for working in this adrenaline-pumped environment. Look for tight-fitting, but beautifully cut shirts in **luxurious fabrics**, but keep them on the right side of professional.

CREATIVE JOB

If your job involves being arty, a splash of colour or an edgy top or jacket can give off the right signals and get you noticed. You need to demonstrate your creativity and eye for **detail** while still looking professional, so choose talking-piece items that say something about your personality, such as a **funky** watch, an eye-catching ring or a quirky handbag. Further up-to-the-minute touches can be added by sporting the latest haircut or wild nails.

MANAGEMENT MATERIAL

If your job involves being in charge, your wardrobe will need to look completely 'together'. Think **sophisticated** rather than high fashion and avoid styles that are too girlie or twee. Spend more on shoes and handbags to help complete your **polished** look. If you spend a lot of the day sitting down, choose suit fabrics that incorporate a bit of stretch to avoid creasing, so you never look crumpled.

Fashion crimes to avoid wherever you work

★ **Skirts that are too short.**
★ **Tops that reveal too much cleavage.**
★ **Crop-tops that show your stomach.**
★ **Dirty shoes or trainers.**
★ **Clothes that haven't been ironed.**
★ **Clothes with dirty marks on.**

TO A **WEDDING**

We've all done it, or know someone who has. . .
I'm talking about wearing something unsuitable
to a wedding. It can be a tricky business: choose
a too-short dress or a plunging neckline and you
can be left feeling uncomfortable and **out-of-place** for the duration of the day. Here are some
tips for getting it right.

Don't try to **upstage the bride**. Never wear white –
just think how you'd feel if someone did the same
at your wedding.

Plan for the weather. If it is being
held on a chilly February morning,
don't think you will get away with a
floating chiffon number. Similarly, if it's
mid-August, you will probably end up
hot and red-faced in a tailored suit.

Think about **footwear**. If the wedding runs straight from
the day into the evening, wear shoes you will be able to
stand in all day to prevent being in agony later on.

If it is a **day-to-evening** affair, choose
an outfit that will see you nicely
through both – for example, a slinky
dress worn under a smart jacket that
can be shed later.

Avoid very pale colours if there is lots of booze involved.
Don't let your day be ruined by food or wine spillages –
stick to vivid colours that can easily be sponged down.

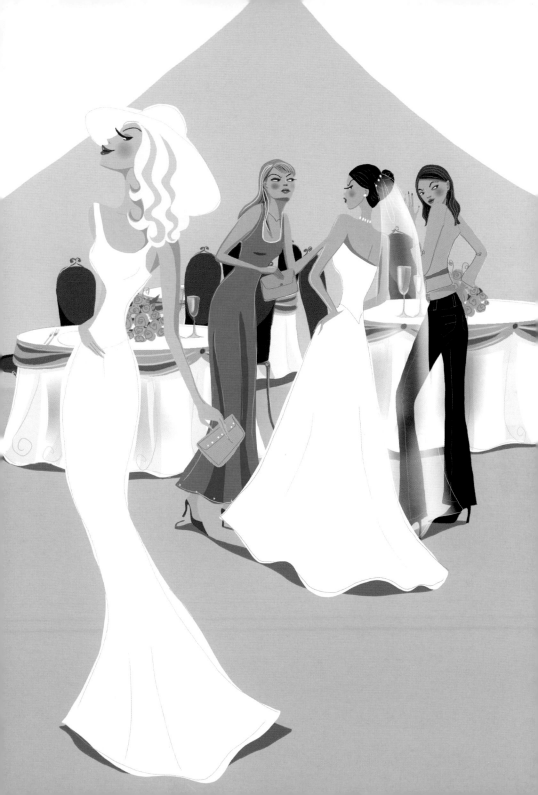

TO **EXERCISE** IN

When it comes to working out, exercise is so much more enjoyable if you know you look good. The problem is, how do you maintain the illusion of **looking cool** and calm while shifting hard-to-burn calories and toning your muscles? Soft, **comfortable fabrics** are one fitness trend that won't ever go out of style. You should choose clothes that work as hard as you do, so look out for fabrics that draw moisture away from your body to keep you dry while you are exercising. Choose **figure-hugging** clothes that allow you to move freely. You need to be able to stretch out in yoga and kick sideways in your body combat class, so go for fabrics that have give and won't restrict movement.

To look good, colour and style are just as important as the fabric of active wear. Having a sexy workout outfit or two can also be another motivator to get you to the gym. Black is a popular choice because it looks good and masks sweat. Add a bit of variety with blues, reds and pinks. If you are planning to exercise outdoors, build up lots of thin layers that can be peeled off as you warm up.

TO **GO OUT**

CRACKING THE DRESS **CODE**

If you've been sent an invite to an evening 'do' take a close look at the wording: careful reading should help avoid outfit **embarrassment**. If you're still not sure what they mean, follow the guide below to understanding partywear lingo.

DRESS: **SMART**

This means you should make an effort but don't turn up frumpy and office-like. A pair of sexy, tailored trousers with a **classy** evening top is smart, as is a special dress. The only real no-no here is jeans.

DRESS: PINK

Don't get carried away. Just because a party has a colour theme, it doesn't mean you have to dress from head-to-foot in that same shade. It is much cooler to acknowledge the theme with a single item, such as a pink skirt. You can even choose to be as low-key as simply wearing **pink nail varnish** or a pink belt.

DRESS: UP

Just to be clear here, this doesn't mean going in fancy dress! It basically means 'put in a **bit of effort**'. This can be as subtle as wearing some sexy high heels or dressing up a top and trousers with some sparkly jewellery. Just don't wear the same outfit you would for a night down the pub.

DRESS: COCKTAIL

This means it is time to pull out your favourite little black dress, or any other colour of show-stopping frock you own. If you've had your eye on a beautiful dress for some time but thought you had nowhere **special enough** to wear it, now is the time to make that purchase. If you really hate dresses, a pair of smart black trousers with high heels and a **glamorous top** will suffice, especially if matched with glitzy jewellery.

DRESS: TO IMPRESS

If you love eye-catching fashion, this is when you can really come into your own. Think red carpet and film premieres and go for the **latest hot looks**. Killer heels are a must, as is well-thought-out hair and make-up. Attention to detail is the key to dressing to impress.

ON A **FIRST DATE**

It can be tricky to know what to wear on that all-important first date. You want to make an impression without overdoing it. If you are looking to wow him, choose something sexy that accentuates your favourite feature, such as a deep V-neck that reveals a hint of cleavage or a split skirt that reveals a flash of shapely leg as you walk. Opt for something **tried-and-tested** that you'd feel just as comfortable wearing out to dinner with your friends. It is worth trying on the outfit the night before. Walk around the house in it and practise sitting down – you will soon know if you are going to feel comfortable in it. Heels are a good way to **add sexiness**, but never wear new shoes or you'll be in agony by the end of the night. Finally, if people always say you look great in a certain colour – wear it!

Be prepared for special invites

Ask yourself, 'What would I wear if I was invited

...to a wedding this weekend?'

...to a party tonight?'

...for a job interview next week?'

...on a date tomorrow night?'

Now make sure you have a fail-safe outfit for each occasion. If you don't, then whatever is missing should be your next clothing investment. Do this every three months, from now on, no matter how busy you are, and you'll always have something to wear for last-minute invites.

GETTING YOUR OFFICE-TO-PARTY LOOK RIGHT

WHAT YOU NEED TO DO THAT MORNING

Wash your hair when you get up and apply body lotion so that your skin is smooth for the evening. To avoid the hassle of taking another outfit out with you, try to wear something that can be dressed up with a few clever accessories. Go to work with a **sparkly top** under your suit and take sheer tights to swap with your thick daytime ones. But remember, what looks good on a night out with the girls (lots of cleavage and acres of legs) is probably not the best look for a night out with work and won't, or shouldn't, impress your boss.

PROBLEMS AND SOLUTIONS

Problem

You don't have space to take a separate pair of party shoes to work, but can't face a whole day wearing killer heels.

Solution

Try some insteps, available from most pharmacies. They will cushion and stabilize your feet, preventing achy feet and back and let you **dance the night away**! They are also cleverly designed to stop your weight tilting backwards, improving your posture so you look slimmer into the bargain.

Problem

Unwanted lumps and bumps.

Solution

Good support underwear is a must to make you look slim and streamlined in your party outfit. Look for an **all-in-one bodysuit** that will flatten your tum, shape your hips and lift your bust.

Problem

Chipped nails.

Solution

Fast-dry polish. Varnished nails make you look instantly more groomed, but can take an age to dry. Solve the problem by using one of the latest **speedy polishes** to paint your nails while you sit at your computer. Most dry in under a minute, so there's no danger of smudging.

Problem

Chunky-looking calves.

Solution

Vaseline. If your legs are bare and you are worried they look too chunky, run a line of Vaseline or **baby oil** along the centre of your shins and calves. As it catches the light it helps to create the **illusion** of slimness.

Christmas party dressing tips

★ Wear a long, warm coat or cloak to cover up until you get to the venue. It will save your dignity on the way and will help you to make a real entrance when you remove it. You will be thankful for it while waiting for a taxi home at the end of the night too!

★ Take a sparkly gold or silver bag and matching sandals – they will add instant glamour to even the most ordinary dress.

★ Wear shoes you can walk and dance in – you will be glad you did by midnight.

★ Avoid anything that will make you feel self-conscious, such as a skirt you have to keep pulling down or a top you need to keep hitching up – you won't be able to relax and will look awkward.

★ Don't wear jewellery you are afraid to lose. Christmas parties are not well known for being sedate and a lost family heirloom will be sure to ruin your night.

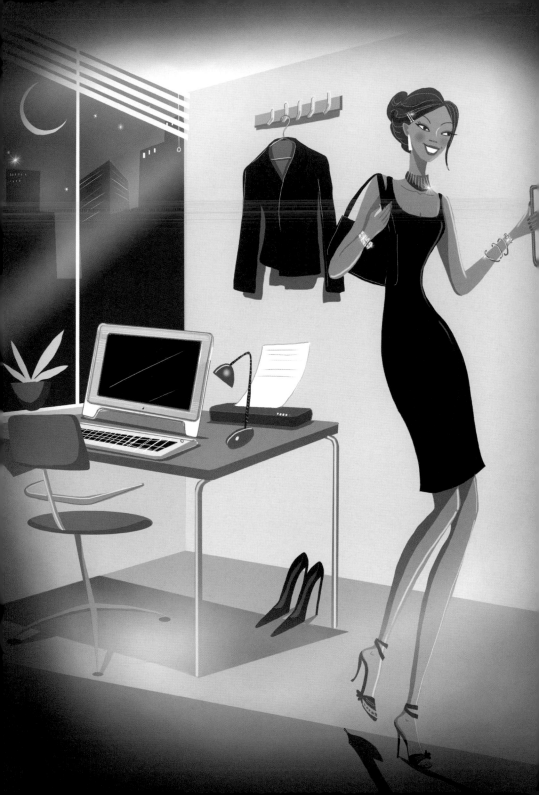

THE LITTLE **BLACK DRESS**

A well-cut little black dress (LBD) is every busy girl's best friend. It is timelessly sexy and, like any true classic, can always be reinvented. Nothing makes flesh look more nude than black, which is what makes it such a **sensual choice** for women. It is worth investing in a dress that looks effortlessly good. Choose a shape that **flatters** your figure: for example, don't wear ultra-thin straps if you hate your arms and avoid Lycra if you have a pot belly.

One of the best things about the LBD is the huge amount of diverse styles you can find on the high street, so whatever the current trend, your budget or taste you can always find something to suit you.

FIVE WAYS TO **WEAR YOUR LBD**

If it is striking, let the dress do all the work. Don't confuse a cutting-edge shape with too many accessories.

Find the **perfect shoes** to go with it. As a rule stick to flats, kitten heels or long boots for daytime and then **vamp it up** with strappy heels by night.

If it is plain and simple, **dress it up**. Try quirky accessories such as a funky belt or a brightly coloured silk scarf.

Deck yourself out in fabulous jewellery. Eye-catching earrings and **big-statement** necklaces can transform the simplest dress into something really special.

Always make a **special effort** with your hair and make-up when wearing an LBD to further its impact.

FIVE WAYS **NOT TO WEAR** YOUR LBD

Don't wear more than two black items in one outfit. Choose handbags or shoes in **brighter** colours.

Never wear the LBD with tights. Bare, freshly shaved and tanned (fake or natural) **legs** look far **sexier**.

Never wear visible **bra straps**. They'll ruin the sophisticated shape of a LBD.

Don't skimp and buy a badly fitting or cheaply made LBD.

Don't wear big baggy white pants under your LBD – it's hard to feel sexy if you're not dressed the part from the inside out. So always wear **slinky black underwear**.

Black out

Classy and stylish, black makes a good base for most wardrobes, which can then be dressed up with brighter colours. Don't be embarrassed if you have a large amount of black in your wardrobe. It is, and always will be, the most stylish of colours.

Black must-haves
- ★ **Winter coat**
- ★ **Classic polo neck**
- ★ **Smart trousers**
- ★ **Knee-length skirt**
- ★ **Boots**
- ★ **Court shoes**
- ★ **Little black dress**

FINDING THE **PERFECT JEANS**

A good-fitting pair of jeans is the ultimate fashion staple. But finding the right pair can sometimes seem impossible. When you consider that jeans are probably the **hardest-working item** in your wardrobe, it is worth spending a bit of time figuring out which style suits your figure, before you part with your hard-earned cash.

IF YOU **HAVE**...
Short legs

Steer clear of cropped cuts, turns-ups, ultra baggy styles or flares – they will all exaggerate shortness. Instead, choose fitted jeans or those with a gentle boot cut to elongate stocky pins. Choose **floor length** and wear them with heels to add a few extra inches.

Long legs

You can get away with pretty much **any shape or style**. Show off long limbs with low rise, straight-leg, tight jeans and roll up the bottoms in the summer for a casual look. Watch out for extra-long versions of standard jeans, which are now made by most manufacturers.

Long back

Avoid jeans that are very low-rise as they will make your upper body look even longer. Wear jeans with a top that just skims your hips to make your body look shorter.

Giving rise?

Jeans have been getting **lower and lower** over the past few years but, unless you are ultra-skinny with a perfectly flat tum, you are better off heading for something with a medium-high waist.

Big hips

Jeans that flare out slightly at the bottom can help **counterbalance** the problem of wide hips. Wearing them lower will also lengthen the body.

Heavy thighs

Stick to darker denim as it **disguises** curves and bumps and avoid denim with a 'worn' effect as this will only emphasize your thighs. Choose men's jeans, which are more generous around the thigh.

Big bottom

Avoid straight legs, which can accentuate a heavy bottom, and **choose loose fits** that kick out slightly from the knee.

How to wear your jeans

Don't get stuck in a groove with your jeans style – here's some ways to work your favourite pair, and adapt them for all occasions.

- ★ **Can't bear to wave goodbye to jeans, but need to look neat and tidy for lunch dates and work? Then team jeans with heels, a navy or black blazer and a white shirt for the smart-casual look.**
- ★ **Rolled-up jeans worn with sandals or flip-flops and a loose-fitting cotton tunic top makes the perfect outfit for lazy summer days.**
- ★ **If you're wearing jeans with heels, the trick is to make sure the hemline skims just above the bottom of the heels.**

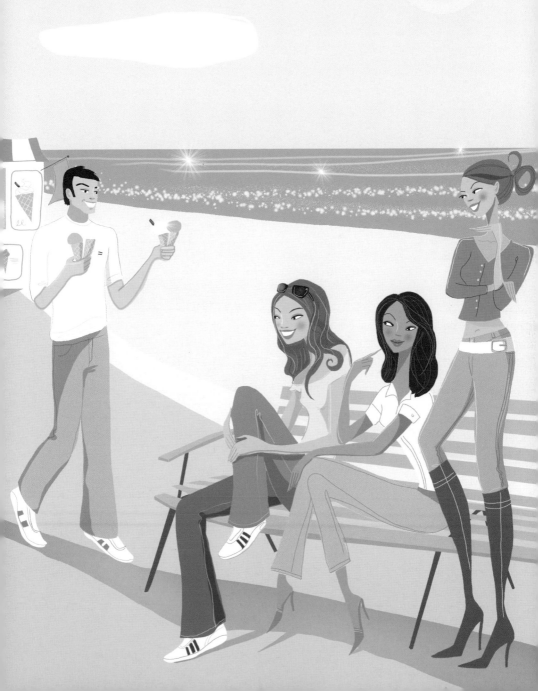

FIVE TIPS FOR JEAN-BUYING SUCCESS,
WHATEVER YOUR SIZE

Choose a good fit

Don't buy jeans just because the size on the label looks good – sizes and cuts vary widely depending on the make. Start with your normal size and don't be reluctant to choose the **next size up** if they don't feel good. A comfortable pair of jeans that fit well will look best on you regardless of the size.

The darker, the better

Unless you are ultra-thin, stay away from very light-coloured or stonewashed jeans. Dark jeans make everyone **look slimmer** and will go with just about anything. They also look more elegant.

Go for the long version

When you go shopping, wear a pair of shoes with heels that are similar to what you usually wear with jeans. Keep in mind that jeans might **shrink**, and when they do, the length can shrink too, so it's better to go with the longer pair. Even preshrunk jeans will shrink when you first wash them, so if you do buy long, always wash them before you have them taken up.

Opt for the boot cut

Stay away from large flare legs that will add bulk. boot-cut jeans have just the right amount of curve at the bottom of the legs to look **stylish** and make your legs appear longer.

Try the **latest fashion**

If you've been dying to try a pair of low-rise hipsters, go ahead. Just make sure you are comfortable wearing them and they aren't so low that you've got **acres of flesh showing** when you bend over!

Keeping jeans in **good shape**

Most denim specialists advise leaving jeans well alone. Washing them too often will cause fading and wear and tear, so only wash them when really necessary – denim is a hardwearing fabric that doesn't get dirty or smelly easily. If you can't bear to do this, however, make sure that when you do wash them it is on a cool cycle and they are turned inside out. The best way to keep dark indigo colours vivid is to wash them in cold water with only a tiny bit of detergent and dry them indoors, rather than on a line outside where they can be faded by the sun. Iron jeans inside out to prevent shiny scorch marks.

★**TIP** Check out the body imagers now available in some department stores and on the internet, where you can discover exactly how different styles and cuts of jeans will look on your individual body shape. For the website versions, you simply type in your dimensions.

THE PERFECT HOLIDAY WARDROBE

Who hasn't lugged a heavy, bulging bag away on holiday, only to bring half the clothes back unworn? To avoid this, you need to learn how to pack only what you need, but still have enough clothes to look great every day of your vacation.

Always start by writing a specific list before you pack – it saves time in the long run and will ensure that you don't forget anything or pack heaps of unnecessary items. **List everything** from shampoo to pants and think in terms of outfits, trying to coordinate everything you pack.

YOUR BASIC HOLIDAY ESSENTIALS
A week by the sea

If you are going on a beach holiday somewhere hot, start with your swimwear, as it is what you will be wearing most of the time. Pack one swimsuit and two bikinis, both in bright, bold colours, and take a few matching **sarongs**, tops and tunics to transform them into outfits. Take a pair of flip-flops and a pair of pretty evening sandals, plus the essential shades and a sun hat. Finally, pack one **versatile** outfit, such as linen trousers and a cotton long-sleeve top that you can wear for shopping or museum visits in air-conditioned buildings.

A **weekend** in the **country**

If it is winter, pack one pair of trousers and one pair of jeans, with two warm sweaters and two evening tops. For your feet take one pair of comfy walking boots and one pair of smarter evening shoes.

If it is summer, pack one pair of cotton trousers with a T-shirt and a lightweight sweater, plus a pretty, strappy top for the evening. Also pack a **summer dress** that is versatile enough to wear day and night and two pairs of sandals, one with flat heels that you can walk around in and one with higher heels for night-time.

A two-day **city break**

Think Audrey Hepburn in Paris – chic and stylish – and you can't go far wrong. Take one pair of trousers or Capri pants with a daytime sweater and an evening top to **dress them up** at night. For the second day, wear a simple dress with flat pumps and pack some killer heels and classy jewellery to transform it into a sexy evening outfit.

Packing **tips**

If you are space-limited, roll up your clothing instead of folding it – it's amazing how small it becomes and, consequently, how much more you will fit in your bag. It will also save you time ironing when you get to your destination.

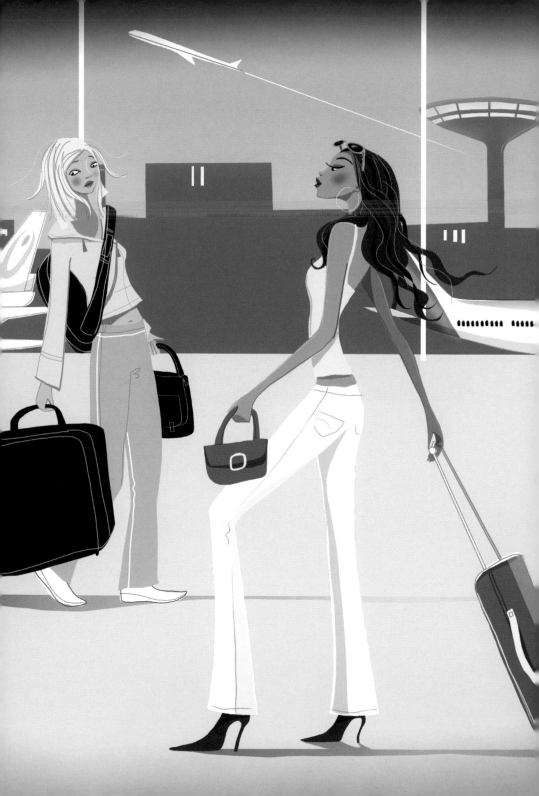

WHAT **KIND OF BAG** TO TAKE

The right kind of bag will save you **time and hassle** at the airport. Here's what to choose and when.

The **hard** line

If you are carrying clothes that need to **look smart** at your destination, or if you have fragile items, a hard suitcase is the answer. Layering carefully folded items with tissue means you won't need to iron them when you unpack. Get a case with wheels to save your neck and back.

Be a **softy**

If you are a busy mother going off for the weekend with a baby in-tow, a big soft holdall is just what you need. The squishiness makes it perfect for squashing into car boots, plus it is **light and durable**. Just don't use it to carry anything breakable or expect clothes to survive without creasing. To avoid crumpled clothes, pack items, like sweaters or cardigans, that are made from such fabrics as jersey or Tactel.

A right **carry-on**

If you are going away for no more than a week and can be disciplined enough with what you pack, a carry-on bag is one of the most **stress-free** ways to travel. Make sure the size and weight match airline rules, which differ from company to company, to avoid the embarrassment of being turned away at the check-in.

Hand luggage

This should be avoided if possible. A small handbag with your passport and purse should be enough. Heavy bags will just become awkward and make travel a lot more arduous.

FANCY **FOOTWORK**

Good shoes are essential – they hold the power to **make or break** an outfit and having the perfect pair of shoes for every outfit will save you many hours of agonizing. Remember, though, not every shape will be flattering, so follow these tips to find out what style will work best for you.

TYPES OF **SHOE**

Strappy sandals

The perfect summer evening shoe, great for slimming legs and more flattering for chunky ankles than closed toes.

Ankle straps

Best avoided unless you have very long, thin legs as they will make your legs look wider and shorter.

Sling-**backs**

This universally flattering shape can be worn by everyone and will smarten up any outfit.

High **heels**

Great for lengthening your legs and making your calves and ankles look shapelier. If you're short, however, don't go for anything higher than two inches or you'll look like you're tottering!

Mules

Ideal for summer daywear as they look good with both trousers and skirts; a mid-heel will suit all shapes and sizes.

D'Orsay **pumps**

These are shoes that have a closed toe and heel, but are bare in-between. They offer a good compromise between sandals and shoes and suit most leg shapes and outfits.

Closed toes

If you hate your feet in strappy sandals, but still want to look glamorous these are the answer. Add a heel and they will look just as 'dressed-up' and sexy.

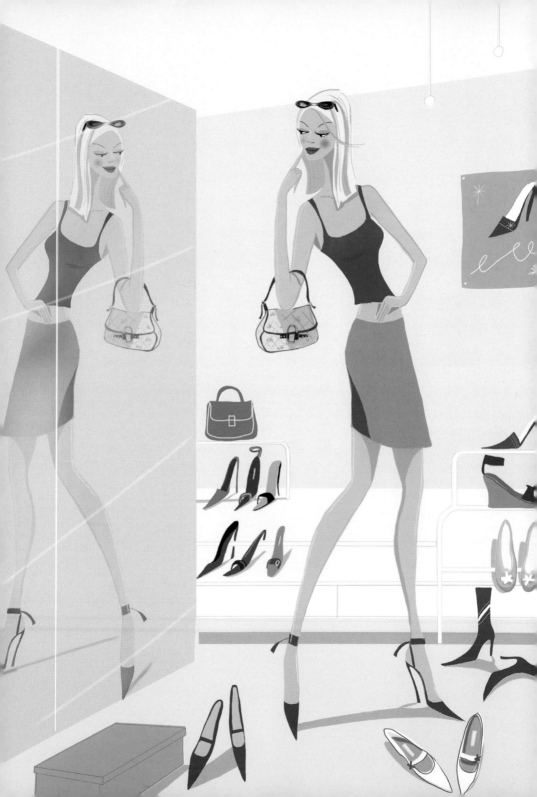

COLOUR

A few pairs of neutral shoes in your wardrobe are always useful, but forget the old rule that shoes have to be black, silver or gold or have to match your handbag. **Matching colours** can be a bit tacky, but your shoes should not be too dark or too light for your outfit. A good rule is to match them to one of the less dominant colours in your outfit, whether it's a swirl of colour in your skirt print or even a bead in your earrings. If your outfit is one colour, don't match your shoes exactly or you could look like a bridesmaid! Instead choose shoes that are in different shades of the same colour. It is generally more flattering if shoes are slightly darker than the outfit.

Vivid colours are an instant way to transform a day outfit into an evening one or add a touch of flair to a sedate dress. Try taking risks. If you like looking edgy you can clash your shoes with your outfit: for example, wearing red shoes with a pink dress. But be warned, it takes **plenty of confidence** to carry it off. Also feet can look bigger in brightly coloured shoes, so opt for neutrals if you hate the size of your tootsies.

COMFORT GUIDE

Remember these pointers when shoe shopping:

- ✿ The thicker the heel tip, the more comfortable and stable the shoes will feel.
- ✿ High heels push your weight forward onto the ball of your foot, so look to see how cushioned this area is.
- ✿ With closed toes, make sure you can still wiggle your toes. If you can't, they are too tight and may cut off your circulation.
- ✿ To get a better idea of how they will fit, always try shoes on towards the end of a shopping trip when your feet are at their hottest and most swollen.

These **boots** were made for **walking!**

Knee-high boots are the ultimate footwear and can be worn with anything. They look great under jeans, with short or long skirts and dresses, so invest in a well-fitting, good-quality leather pair and they will last and last.

PUTTING YOUR BEST FOOT FORWARD

Six foot faux pas to avoid:

Your outfit is very dark but your **shoes are light** and vice versa.

Wearing **open-toed sandals** with chipped or unkempt toenails. If you are going to expose your feet, give yourself a pedicure and paint your nails the night before.

Wearing **worn-out, dirty** or in-desperate-need-of-a-polish shoes. It will completely ruin your look.

Waiting until the last minute to get your shoes heeled. You are likely to do **permanent damage** to the shoe by scuffing the leather base.

Wearing **tights with sandals**. Most fashion experts agree there is nothing worse, so plan ahead and shave or wax your legs and apply fake tan the night before.

Bare legs in winter. Showing off bare white pins looks nasty and, for work, unprofessional, so invest in lots of pairs of funky patterned tights.

Shoe maintenance

★ Put together a simple shoe repair kit that contains polish for every colour of shoe you wear, a protector spray for suede and nubuck, a suede brush and trainer whitener.

★ Clean and polish all your shoes once a month to make sure that they look presentable whenever you need them. At the same time, check if any need to be resoled or reheeled.

★ Choose a shoe repair outlet that also does dry cleaning so you can get both chores done at once.

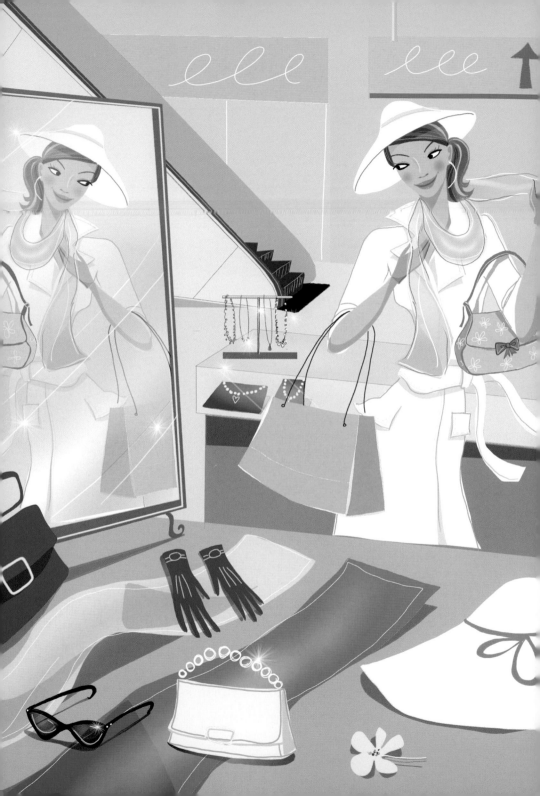

MAKING ACCESSORIES WORK FOR YOU

Your accessory drawer is your box of tricks for updating a look or **transforming** an otherwise boring outfit. Stock it with plenty of inexpensive belts, scarves and jewellery, buying a few new bits each season, and you will always look modern. You should also make sure you have a good collection of day and evening bags to suit any occasion. The trick is to have a host of items that can transform your look with minimum time and fuss, but creating maximum impact. Here's how to add a bit of **glamour** and style without overdosing.

- ✿ Make sure accessories are in **scale** with you – huge items can dwarf smaller women, while tiny, delicate ones can make a tall or large person look bigger.
- ✿ Team intricate, flashy earrings and belts with streamlined, simple outfits.
- ✿ Use accessories to draw **attention** to a part of your body that you like, such as your eyes or waist.
- ✿ Short of cash? Before you buy a new outfit for a special occasion, see if an existing favourite can be **dressed up** with funky accessories.
- ✿ Never over-accessorize – for **maximum impact** stick to one or two items at a time.
- ✿ Invest in a few plain coloured silk and wool **pashminas** – they look far better over evening dresses, winter or summer, than a bulky jacket.

TEN WAYS TO TRANSFORM A LOOK IN SECONDS

Slip a shimmery top under a suit
Even the dullest office clothes can be transformed into a look you can dance the night away in when paired with a **glittery camisole** or halterneck.

Bead it
Adding a **flash of beads** will jazz up the most boring outfit. Invest in a few beaded or sequinned accessories, such as purses, belts and necklaces, and keep them in your drawer at work to add sparkle if you need to go out for an impromptu after-work do.

Fake it
Diamonds add instant glamour, but if you can't afford the real thing, **costume jewellery** looks just as good. Hold your hair up with a diamanté slide or pin a brooch to your top.

Wrap it up
A beautiful shawl or pashmina adds instant sophistication. Embroidered, chiffon styles look great with simple strapless dresses while **chunkier knits** smarten up jeans and boots.

Choose the perfect bag
The choice is endless but suede is great for daytime while **gold or silver** leather add evening chic.

Slip on sexy shoes to vamp up a look
Wear them with everything from trousers to little **black dresses**.

Match dangly **earrings** with an 'up-do'

Off-the-neck hair with earrings will change the way an outfit looks. Hoops and **vintage beaded** earrings go with most clothes and provide an interesting focal point for otherwise simple looks.

Add a **hat**

Nothing attracts attention like a hat. It takes confidence to wear one, so choose **classic shapes** such as a fedora or beret to make the look easier to pull off.

Pick the right **shades**

A great pair of sunglasses will add an air of **movie-star glamour** and look stylish even worn on top of your head.

Don a **blazer**

This will smarten up plain black trousers or jeans and add class to **simple white** shirts.

Mixing gold and silver

Jewellery etiquette used to dictate that silver and gold should never be worn together but this has changed in recent years. If you are after a more traditional, classic look it is still best to keep them separate, but if you are trying to create something a bit more edgy, mixing metals can work well. Many jewellery designers are now making rings and bracelets that mix gold and silver together in one piece, which means it is easier to mix and match them with other items.

QUICK, CALL THE FASHION POLICE!

Even the most stylish of us make mistakes from time to time. Here's how to avoid the worst of them.

YOUR CLOTHES ARE TOO TIGHT

We have all squeezed into a size smaller than we really are – it makes us feel slimmer to say, 'I got into a 10!' when really a 12 would have been more comfortable. However, there is nothing guaranteed to make you **look bigger** than too-tight clothes. Always wear your 'real' size – no one else will know what it is.

YOUR CLOTHES ARE TOO LOOSE

Another common mistake is to wear baggy clothes to try and hide excess weight, but be warned – this simply **adds more pounds**. Instead of covering everything up, accentuate your positive points and show off your curves. Fitted tops and trousers are far more **flattering** than over-sized tent-like dresses.

YOU ARE MIXING TOO MANY STYLES

Don't make the mistake of trying to satisfy everything that is currently in fashion in one outfit – you run the risk of looking **ridiculous** and like you are trying too hard.

YOU HAVEN'T IRONED YOUR CLOTHES

What's the point of spending hours choosing the perfect outfit only to put it on unironed? No clothes look good wrinkled, no matter how expensive they are, so always keep a good **steam iron** handy. If you really hate ironing, buy clothes made from fabrics that don't wrinkle as much. If you are away from home and have no iron, hang up clothes in the bathroom, as the steam from the bath and shower will help the creases to drop out. If all else fails and you can afford it, pay someone else to do your washing and ironing so you never have to worry about them again!

YOUR **UNDERWEAR** IS SHOWING

A great outfit can be ruined by visible underwear, so invest in some well-fitting, **streamlined** smalls. If your underwear still shows, your trousers or skirt are probably too tight.

TOO MANY **PRINTS**

Don't try to mix and match prints or your look will end up being far too busy. Choose a pattern on **either the top or bottom** but not both. And remember, patterns don't look good on everyone, even if you are one of those people who look good in just about anything.

THE **WRONG** ACCESSORIES

Top off your look with accessories that match your style. Choose the correct length necklace to suit the **neckline** of your top or dress. Short chains and chokers tend to make your neck appear larger and never, ever wear necklaces over the top of sweaters!

YOUR SKIRT'S **TOO SHORT**

It might look sexy, but if you don't feel **comfortable** you will be continuously trying to tug the hemline down. As a test, make sure you can **sit down** without having to worry about what parts of your body you are exposing.

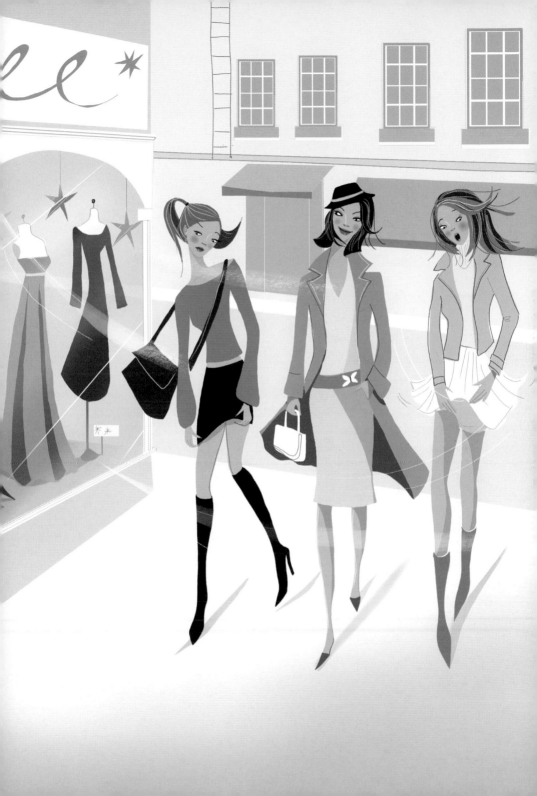

QUICK TIPS TO GUARANTEE A **GOOD** FIT

Save hours in front of the mirror at home by getting the **perfect fit** every time you buy something.

- ✿ Always check the fit of what you are about to buy in a **three-way mirror**, so you can see it from every angle.
- ✿ Always sit down in a garment when trying it on. What may fit beautifully when you are standing can pull or **gape** open once you sit down.
- ✿ Similarly, have a walk in it. Many skirts and dresses can look perfect when standing still, only to **ride up** when you walk along.
- ✿ The waistband of your skirt should **not pucker** or roll up.
- ✿ Sleeves of jackets and coats should just hit the wrist.
- ✿ Fabric should not cling to or stretch over problem areas, so never wear anything too tight.
- ✿ Don't put off making wardrobe choices until you have lost weight. Choose pieces that can **camouflage** problem areas instead.
- ✿ Invest in **alterations**. Clothing that doesn't fit will never leave your wardrobe.
- ✿ Forget about fashion. Find the **hem length** that is most **flattering** to you and stick with it!

Five fashion items to avoid
at all costs

1 Mid-calf boots

Unless you are very tall, they tend to 'cut' legs in half, making them look short and a little stumpy.

2 Crop tops

These should only be worn by those under 18 or with washboard abs. Even skinny girls often find they have a 'roll' when they sit down in a crop.

3 Any animal prints

These always look tacky and cheap and never classy, even when a top designer makes the item.

4 Drainpipe jeans

These only suit those blessed with supermodel proportions (endless legs, a tiny bottom, super-skinny thighs and no hips). Need I say more?

5 White trousers

These can look terrible unless you are slim, so only wear them if they are loose-fitting and made from a good-quality fabric that is not see-through and it's the height of summer.

DISASTERS EN ROUTE AND
HOW TO FIX THEM FAST

YOU'VE SNAGGED YOUR TIGHTS
What to do

Always carry clear **nail polish** in your handbag. Painted on, it will stop any runs in their tracks.

Prevention tactic

When you buy your tights, make sure they are the correct size. Too small and they are more likely to ladder so always go for the **large size**.

YOUR DEODORANT HAS LEFT
WHITE MARKS ON YOUR DARK TOP
What to do

Most deodorant marks can be gently sponged off with plenty of warm water.

Prevention tactic

Use an antiperspirant that is specifically designed not to leave behind marks on your clothes.

SOMEONE HAS SPILT RED WINE ON YOUR WHITE OUTFIT
What to do

Ask the barman or party host for **soda water** or **white wine**. These are the best liquids for gently sponging off a red wine stain.

Prevention tactic

Don't wear white. Play safe and stick to black at parties where the alcohol is flowing freely!

YOU'VE SAT IN **CHEWING GUM**
What to do

Remove as much of the gum as possible with a knife and then hold an **ice cube** to the stain until it hardens. You should then be able to scrape off the remainder. Finally, sponge the area with hot water.

Prevention tactic

Always look down at seats before sitting on them!

YOUR CAT'S LEFT **HAIR** ALL OVER YOUR **BLACK COAT**
What to do

If you don't have a clothes brush handy, **masking tape** will work just as well. Wrap a strip over your hand and use it to pick off the stray hairs.

Prevention tactic

If this is a frequent problem, carry a mini roll of tape in your handbag at all times, or **shave the cat**!

YOU'VE GOT **RAIN MARKS** ON NEW SUEDE
What to do

Gently rub the marks with a nail file, being very careful not to damage the suede. This should ease out the stains.

Prevention tactic

Invest in a suede **protector spray** and spray a layer over your shoes or jacket every couple of weeks.

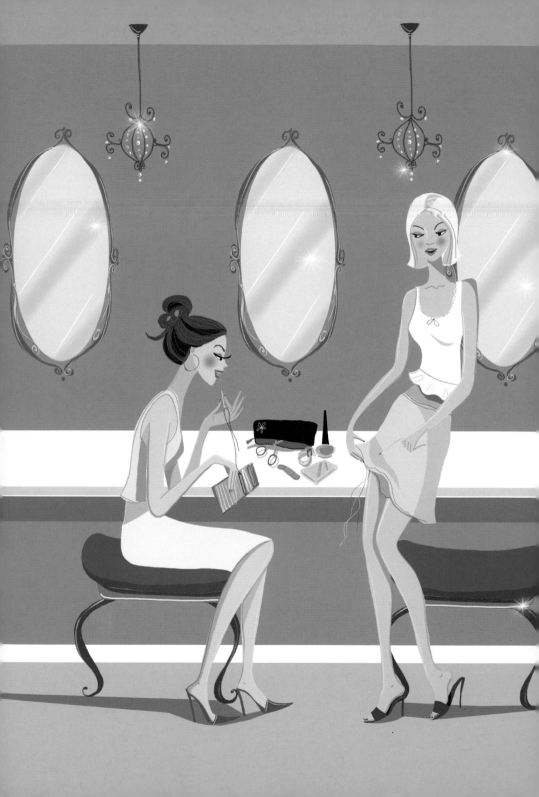

YOUR **HEEL** HAS BROKEN
What to do

Stop at a heel bar and see if there is anything that can be done to rescue it. Failing that, you will have to stop at the nearest shoe shop and buy a new pair of shoes.

Prevention **tactic**

Stick to flats if you have to walk any distance and always keep a **spare pair** of shoes at work for emergencies like this.

YOUR HANDBAG **STRAP SNAPS**
What to do

Rescue the strap by knotting it back onto the bag until it can be **restitched**. If it is not salvageable, cut off the other strap and carrying it as a hand-held purse until it can be replaced.

Prevention **tactic**

Be careful not to overload your handbag as extra strain may cause the strap to snap. **Clear it out** once a week to make sure you are not carrying around lots of junk you don't actually need.

★**TIP** Make your handbag a mini quick-fix kit that can cope with any emergency. Stocking it with a small bottle of clear nail polish, a tiny roll of tape, a nail file, a mini pair of scissors and a spare pair of tights should cover most eventualities.

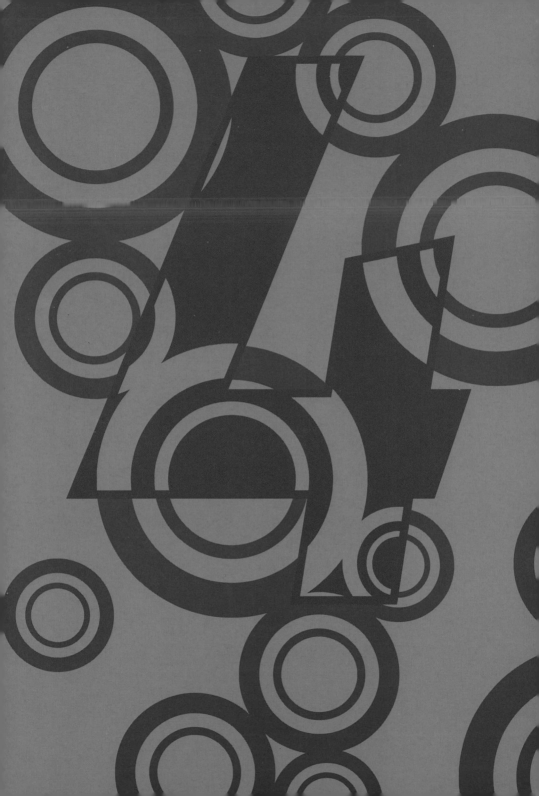

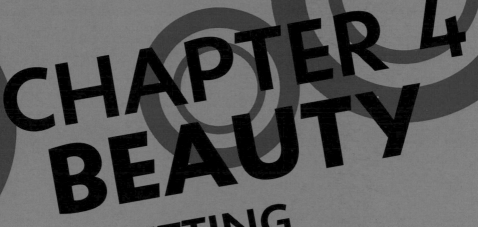

CHAPTER 4
BEAUTY

GETTING GORGEOUS – FAST!

And now for the cosmetic touches to complete every busy girl's transformation – how to look **fabulous** in a flash. Get ready for your hair, make-up and skincare dilemmas to be solved and sorted.

Do you find you're always **rushing** from work to a party or from dinner with the family to meet friends? Always being on the go doesn't leave a girl much time to get her hair and make-up just right. Luckily, looking good doesn't have to take hours to accomplish. With a few **clever tricks** – even when you have a frantic schedule of work, friends and fitness – you can get yourself looking **glam** and **gorgeous** in no time.

So whether you've got an impromptu date or are having a manic morning scramble to get ready, the **beauty tips** here will leave you looking pretty – pronto. And you'll never have one of those 'too busy to be beautiful' moments again!

You'll learn how to identify your skin type and the best way to look after it, how to create the **perfect face** in next to no time at all, and tips on streamlining your make-up bag and discarding unnecessary products so it contains only the essentials. Plus you'll find **solutions** for fixing common beauty disasters in seconds and ways to transform your face for a date or last-minute party.

The advice in this section will also provide tips on giving yourself an effective home facial, whipping up face masks in minutes from a few kitchen fridge staples, and salon-perfect **mini manicures** – all designed to save you time and money while leaving you sensationally stunning-looking and well groomed.

WHAT SKIN TYPE ARE YOU?

Having good skin is the very foundation of looking your best, but as all busy girls know, a hectic lifestyle can leave little time for pore pampering. The first key to **speedy skincare** is to understand what kind of skin you have so you know what products to use on it and how to quickly combat any problems that may arise. If you are not sure how to define your skin, take this mini quiz to find out.

Q1 HOW DOES YOUR SKIN FEEL IF YOU WASH YOUR FACE WITH SOAP AND WATER?

A Tight and uncomfortable.

B Smooth and comfortable.

C Dry and itchy in places.

D Fine, quite comfortable.

E Dry in some areas and smooth in others.

Q2 HOW DOES YOUR SKIN FEEL IF YOU CLEANSE IT WITH A CREAM-BASED CLEANSER?

A Relatively comfortable.

B Smooth and comfortable.

C Sometimes comfortable, sometimes itchy.

D Oily all over.

E Oily in some areas and smooth in others.

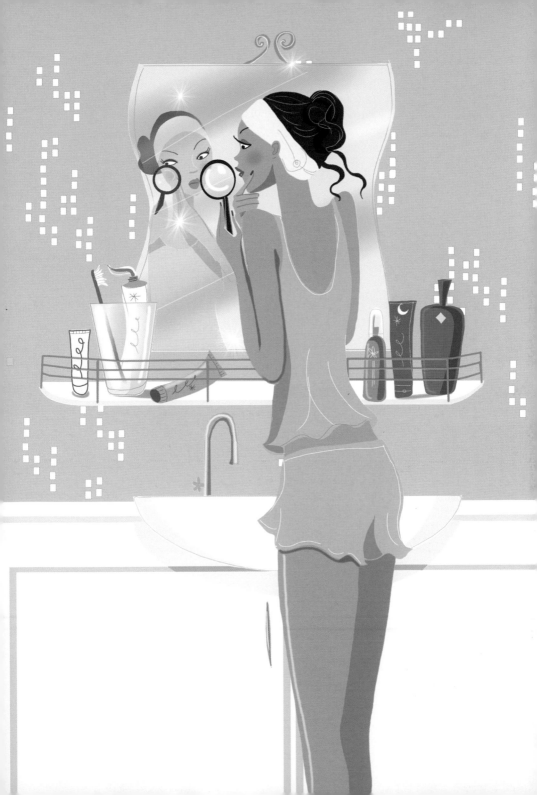

**Q3 HOW DOES YOUR SKIN NORMALLY
LOOK BY LUNCHTIME?**

A Flaky and dry.

B Fresh and clean.

C Flaky patches with some redness.

D Shiny everywhere.

E Shiny across the T-zone only.

Q4 HOW OFTEN DO YOU BREAK OUT IN SPOTS?

A Hardly ever.

B Only just before your period.

C Occasionally.

D Often and everywhere.

E Often, but only across the T-zone.

**Q5 HOW DOES YOUR SKIN REACT
WHEN YOU USE A FACIAL TONER?**

A It stings.

B It is fine.

C It stings and itches.

D It feels fresh and clean.

E It feels fresher in some areas,
but stings in others.

Q6 HOW DOES YOUR SKIN REACT TO A RICH NIGHT CREAM?

A It feels very comfortable.

B It feels comfortable.

C Sometimes it feels comfortable, other times it feels irritated.

D It feels really greasy.

E It feels oily on the T-zone, but comfortable on the cheeks.

MOSTLY 'A'S – **DRY SKIN**

Your skin is prone to flakiness and never feels comfortable unless you have just applied moisturizer. It has a 'parched' look, caused by its **inability to retain moisture**, and often feels tight. Its dryness is exacerbated by the wind, extremes of temperature and air-conditioning. Without **careful care**, this type of skin is prone to premature ageing.

What to do

- ❀ Don't use tap water or soap on your skin – they are both too drying. Use a rich cold cream to cleanse instead.
- ❀ Massage with moisturizing oil or serum every night to help stimulate the sebaceous glands into producing more oil.
- ❀ Be generous with eye cream in the areas surrounding the eyes, where tiny lines can begin to form.

MOSTLY 'B'S – **NORMAL SKIN**

Your skin has an even tone and a soft, smooth texture with no visible pores or blemishes, and no greasy patches or flaky areas. This type of skin is neither greasy nor dry. It **glows with health**, which stems from good blood circulation. You may get the odd pimple just before you menstruate, due to increased hormonal activity, but they soon clear up. However, your skin still needs to be cared for. Neglect can lead to signs of premature ageing and wrinkling.

What to do

- ❀ The only care this skin requires is cleansing twice a day with a gentle facial wash and water, and toning with something mild, such as rose water.
- ❀ Use a light moisturizer with an SPF of at least 15 every day to keep your skin protected from the sun's damaging UV rays.
- ❀ Once a week, boost circulation and smooth the surface of the skin with a tightening or moisturizing face mask.

MOSTLY 'C'S – **SENSITIVE SKIN**

Your skin is thin and fine-textured. It reacts quickly to both heat and cold, which means it is **prone to dryness** and sunburn. It is commonly dry, delicate and prone to allergic reactions. The upper skin layers and certain detergents and cosmetics can cause irritation, leaving the skin red and blotchy.

What to do

✿ Apply a **sunscreen** every day to protect the skin from environmental damage. Select one designed for sensitive skin and with an SPF of 30.

✿ Choose products that are free from perfume, colours and other possible allergens. Look for the word '**hypoallergenic**' on the bottle. People with specific allergies should always check the ingredients, however, as hypoallergenic only means that it has undergone some level of skin testing – it does not mean you will not be allergic to the cream.

✿ Wash with a **light cleansing milk** that can be removed with cotton wool, as water can be irritating to your skin.

★**TIP** If you're booking a facial, make sure you let the therapist know you have sensitive skin and mention any products or ingredients that caused, or seemed to cause, reactions previously.

MOSTLY 'D'S – **OILY SKIN**

Your skin is shiny with large pores and is prone to blackheads and pimples. In this type of skin, the oil-producing sebaceous glands are overactive and produce **more oil than is needed**. This can be hereditary and may be made worse by pregnancy, taking certain contraceptive pills, or high levels of stress – all of which trigger more oil production. On the positive side, however, the great advantage of oily skin is that it **ages at a slower rate** than other skin types.

What to do

✿ Oily skin needs **gentle cleansing** with soap or a foaming wash to remove surface oil. But avoid harsh products that strip your skin of oil because this simply causes the oil glands to work overtime to compensate for the loss of natural oils.

✿ Use **oil-free moisturizers** to maintain a shine-free complexion.

✿ Use a deep-cleansing **clay-based mask** once or twice a week to help prevent blackheads.

✿ Choose cosmetics and skincare products that are specifically designed for oily skin and say '**noncomedogenic**' on the bottle, as this means they have been tested to make sure they don't block pores and trigger the formation of blemishes.

★**TIP** Don't avoid sunscreen for fear of adding too much oil to your skin – you'll regret the sun damage in the future. Simply choose a light gel or lotion that is specifically for oily skin.

MOSTLY 'E'S – COMBINATION

Your skin is a combination of both oily and dry. It has a greasy, **T-shaped panel** consisting of your nose, forehead and chin, but your cheeks and the area around the eyes are prone to dryness. This type of skin is very common and it should be treated as if it were two different types of skin.

What to do

- ✿ Use a **light cleansing lotion** that is moisturizing enough to **soothe** the cheek area, but also effective in removing oil from the T-zone.
- ✿ Use a mildly astringent **toner** on the T-zone, avoiding the cheeks.
- ✿ Apply a **light moisturizer** to the cheeks only and use an eye cream to help prevent fine lines.

Good skincare maintenance

★ To help your skin stay in tip-top condition and keep problems to a minimum, try to go for a regular, monthly facial – it will really make a difference to the condition of your skin. The therapist will also be able to help assess your skin type and advise you on home care and any seasonal skin changes.

★ At home, set aside 30 minutes a week for a mini home facial – while you are waiting for the bath to fill up is a good time. Start by cleansing and then exfoliate, using the correct product for your skin type. Apply a suitable mask for the recommended time, then wash off and moisturize. Following this simple regime should help to keep skin soft and clear between facials.

★ Take a daily multivitamin to feed your skin from within and help keep it healthy. You can buy specific vitamins that are designed to boost 'skin, hair and nails'. They contain the correct balance of vitamins, minerals and antioxidants to keep your skin looking and feeling healthy.

YOUR DIY FACIAL PLAN

Do you ever have to cancel an appointment for a facial to meet a work deadline or catch up with a friend? Don't worry. With all the high-tech products on the market these days, you can now get salon-like results in the **comfort** of your **own home**. In addition to your weekly mini facial, try this 60-minute intensive treatment once a month.

LATHER UP

Before you begin, carefully take off any eye make-up using gentle eye make-up remover and cotton wool. Then, massage a gentle, **foaming cleanser** into your skin for about a minute, using upwards, circular strokes. Focus on areas that are prone to congestion, such as your forehead and around the nose. This step will remove make-up and surface grime. Rinse, then repeat the process – double cleansing is a salon trick that guarantees really clean skin.

SCRUB-A-DUB DUB

Proper exfoliation makes every product, from masks to moisturizers, work more effectively. Skin treatments are better able to penetrate your skin when they are not prevented from doing so by dead surface cells. Choose a scrub made from fine, spherical particles and rub it into your skin with outward, circular motions, then rinse. **Be gentle** – the idea is to leave your skin **soft**, not red raw! If your skin is sensitive, choose a cream exfoliate that contains fruit acids. These great products can just be left on the skin to work like a mask and are nonabrasive.

★**TIP** Never use a body scrub on your face. The particles will be too coarse and could damage delicate facial skin.

MASK IT

Face masks these days serve many purposes and can treat a whole host of different skin problems. For oily skin there is the classic clay variety, which absorbs grease and helps to **unblock pores**. Gel or cream masks are perfect for adding moisture to dehydrated skins, while cooling and anti-inflammatory ones will soothe sensitive skin. If you have combination skin, simply apply a clay mask across the forehead and a moisturizing mask on the cheeks.

After your mask has been on for the advised length of time, rinse it off thoroughly. Then tone using a gentle, alcohol-free toner. And finally, **lock in all those skin benefits** with a vitamin-rich moisturizer that suits your skin type. Try to schedule your DIY facial so that it finishes just before bedtime. This way you won't have to apply make-up to your newly cleansed skin and it will have a chance to absorb all the nutrients you have applied overnight, so you wake up with a fresh, glowing complexion.

Home spa

Giving yourself the home 'spa' treatment is an excellent way to attend to your beauty needs. Devoting even just one hour to looking after your whole body from head to toe will not only make you feel more groomed and gorgeous, but will help you destress too.

* **Create a salon-like atmosphere with lit candles, an aromatherapy burner or incense, and quiet new-age music.**
* **Adjust the phone volume to low and let your answerphone take all the calls.**
* **Add relaxing aromatherapy oils or foaming oil to the bath water.**
* **Start with a body brush or scrub, apply a hair mask and face mask (or an ice mask), and lie back and relax for 20 minutes.**
* **Afterwards, while your skin is still soft from the soak, tweeze brows and give yourself a manicure (see also pages 306–7).**

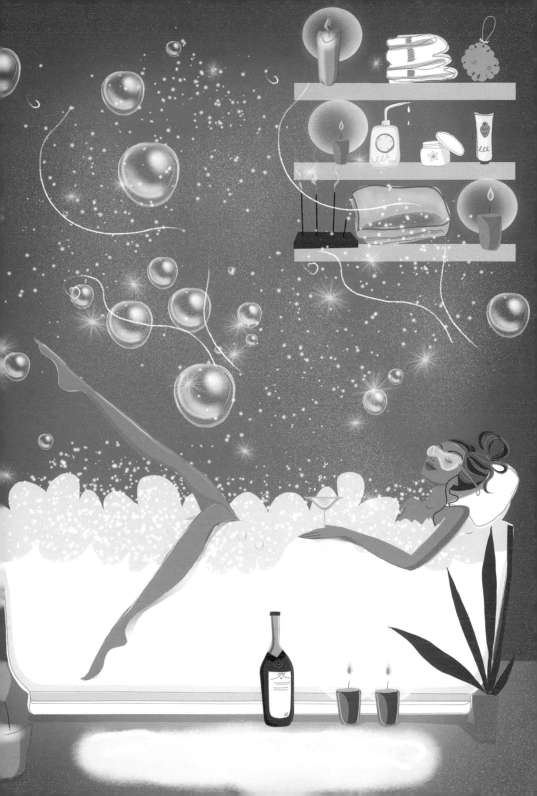

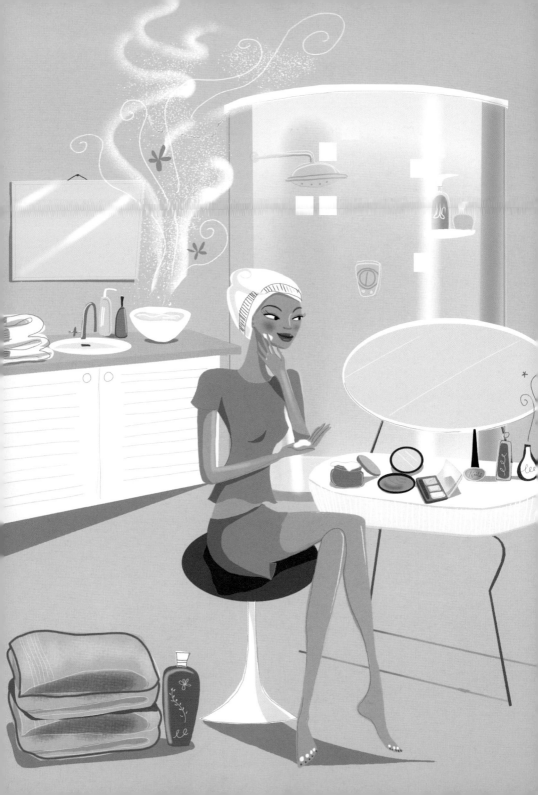

GET **STEAMY**

Steaming your skin will take the cleansing process one stage deeper. It allows the skin to sweat out toxins, one of its natural functions, thus helping to **cleanse** from the inside out.

Be careful not to hold your face too close to the steam as this may cause broken capillaries. Steaming can also dehydrate your skin – when water evaporates from your face it can take away some of your skin's own moisture – so to prevent this, apply a thin **layer of moisturizer** before hitting the heat. If your skin is very sensitive, limit steam time to the exposure your face gets in your daily hot shower – it is far gentler.

1 Fill a bowl with hot water and sprinkle in a few drops of **essential oil** – tea tree oil is good for oily skin, rose soothes delicate or mature skin and lavender is great for all skin types. (Always check with a registered aromatherapist or pharmacist if you are pregnant as some oils can be harmful.)

2 Place a towel over the back of your head, lean your face over the bowl and bring the towel down around it. Steam for **5 minutes**.

3 Steaming will soften any oil plugs, such as blackheads, that are blocking **pores**. To remove them, wrap both fingertips in tissue and press either side, gently wiggling the area, until the blackhead eases out.

KITCHEN **FRIDGE CURES**

Haven't had enough time to stock up on beauty products but your skin is in desperate need of some serious **pampering**? Then head for your fridge or store cupboard where you'll find a whole host of skin treats that are good enough to eat! Best of all, they are natural and free from nasty additives or perfume. Try some of these to restore a healthy skin tone in no time.

BANANA MASK
A **conditioning** mask that is good for normal skin.

Ingredients
One ripe banana.
One tablespoon of natural yogurt.
One tablespoon of honey.

How to make it
Mash up the banana and mix with the yogurt and honey. Apply to your skin and leave on for 10–15 minutes before washing off to reveal soft, glowing skin.

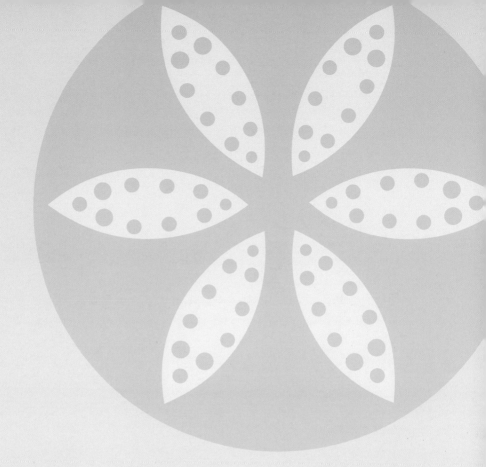

CUCUMBER EYE MASK

A **soothing** mask to brighten the delicate eye area
 – great after a late night.

Ingredients

Half a cucumber.
One tablespoon of natural yogurt.

How to **make** it

Grate the cucumber flesh and mix it with the yogurt.
Make two tea bag-like parcels using kitchen roll and leave
them in the fridge for about 5 minutes. Then remove them
and place one over each eye. Finally, lie back and simply
relax for 10 minutes.

TOMATO MASK

This is an **astringent** mask that is ideal for balancing oily skin.

Ingredients
One ripe tomato.
One tablespoon of natural yogurt.

How to make it
Mash up the tomato and mix it with the yogurt. Apply to the skin and leave for 10 minutes. Don't use this if your skin is sensitive, as the acidic juice of tomatoes can irritate delicate skins.

HONEY MASK

A rich, **nourishing** mask that is good for dry skin.

Ingredients
Two egg yolks.
Two tablespoons of honey.
One teaspoon of almond oil.

How to make it
Blend the egg yolks, honey and almond oil together. Pat on to your face and let it dry for 10 minutes. Rinse off for amazingly soft skin.

MORNING SKINCARE **ROUTINE**

If you're really pushed for time in the mornings adopt a simple, **stress-free** skincare routine.

1 Make **cleansing** your priority and go for a face wash or cleanser that is light and quick. Choose one with skin-soothing ingredients that help banish morning blotches and puffiness.

2 Skip the toner and only use **moisturizer** where it is needed on the face.

3 **Zap blemishes** with a quick application of tea tree oil directly on the spot.

4 If you really have no time for facials and even a 15-minute mask is pushing it, opt for the latest fast-activating products. Many skincare ranges now have **speedy treatments**, such as masks and exfoliate creams, that only need to be left on for 2–3 minutes to work – just enough time to iron your top as you get ready to go out!

QUICK **SKIN RESCUES**

We have all woken up and had those 'aaarghh' moments after seeing ourselves in the mirror. Here's how to combat some of the worst **bad skin moments**, in minutes.

A **LARGE BLEMISH**

Do not attack it with your fingers – it will only make matters worse. Instead hold an ice cube to it for a minute to reduce any swelling, dab on some antiseptic **tea tree oil** with a cotton bud (cotton swab), cover with a little concealer and leave well alone!

PUFFY EYES

Usually the signs of a late night. Don't make the mistake of trying to hide them with lots of make-up. Instead, apply a cold compress or **eye mask** for 5 minutes, then use a thin layer of light-reflecting concealer to brighten the area.

FLAKY LIPS

Take an old toothbrush, dip it in Vaseline or lip balm and gently rub your lips in a circular motion to remove all the dry, flaky bits. Wipe off and then apply another layer of Vaseline for a super-soft pout.

DULL SKIN

Whip out the face exfoliate and gently scrub away any excess skin cells. Follow with a skin **brightening serum** to tighten skin, boost circulation and give you a healthy glow. Finally, add a touch of pink cream blush to the apples of your cheeks.

BLOTCHY PATCHES

Apply a soothing mask for 10 minutes. Choose one that doesn't set and contains **anti-inflammatory ingredients** such as raspberry leaf, camomile and calendula, which will help tone down the redness. Once you have removed the mask, use a thin layer of tinted moisturizer to even out your skin tone.

SUNBURN

Take an aspirin to reduce the inflammation and apply a **soothing after sun lotion** all over the skin – choose one containing aloe vera extract for maximum comfort. Don't try and cover the redness with foundation, just use a little tinted moisturizer and bronzer to even it out. Prevention is always better than cure, so be sure to slather on a high SPF next time you go out.

SHINY T-ZONE

A fast fix for this is to blot with a tissue or blotting sheet and then apply a fine layer of **mattifying loose powder**, using a large brush to sweep off the excess.

HOW TO **SAVE POST-PARTY** SKIN

Late nights, too many cocktails, and not enough water all spell disaster for your complexion. You look in the mirror the next morning, only to find puffiness, dark circles, dry flaky skin, and some hin red spots – **what do you do**?

✿ The main problem you will be facing is dehydrated skin. For an instant boost, **quench your skin's thirst** with a moisturizing mask. Use it all over the face, including the eyelids, and leave on for as long as possible before applying your make-up.

✿ If you can remember, and are in a fit state, try and slather on **extra moisturizer** when you fall into bed after a late night – it will be worth the extra effort when your skin looks great in the morning.

✿ When it comes to concealing the ravages of the night before, most people make the mistake of putting on too much make-up in a bid to hide their skin. This can, however, make it look much worse. Instead, keep things **light and natural**. Go for bright, light-reflecting products that will give your face a healthy glow.

✿ Use a sheer under-eye **concealer** to take the edge off the dark circles and wear lots of lip gloss, rather than lipstick that will only crack on dehydrated lips.

✿ If time (and your boss!) allows, pop into a salon near work during your lunch-break for a **mini facial** to give skin the ultimate morning-after perk up.

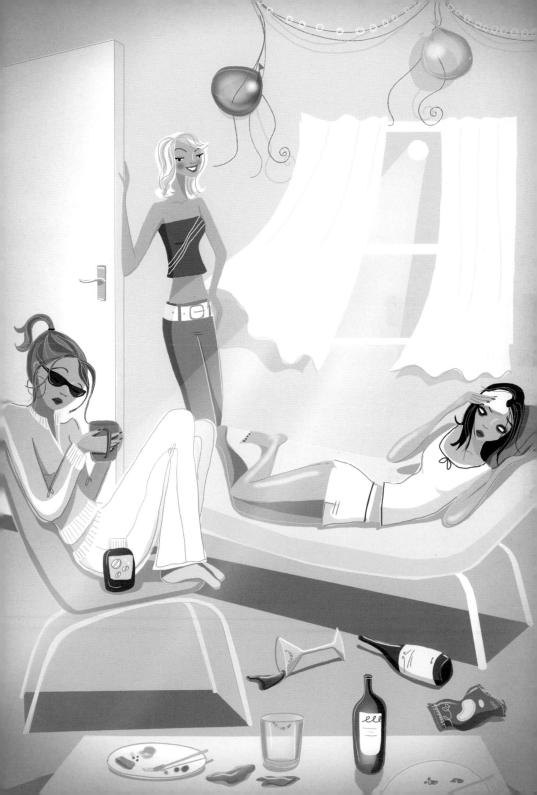

YOUR ESSENTIAL
MAKE-UP KIT

Busy girls need to adopt a minimalist approach to make-up in order to save them valuable time. Here are the only **ten products** you'll ever need, so pare down your beauty bag for a fast routine that will leave you looking fabulous.

Foundation

Choose a medium coverage product that suits your skin type. Some beauty companies will mix a shade just for you to create the **perfect colour**. It costs a little more but it is well worth the expense. And remember, you don't have to wear foundation all over your face, every day. Only use what you need and if your skin looks good, save time and skip it.

Concealer

Buy a colour one shade **lighter** than your skin and use a clean lipstick brush to cover dark shadows, spots and other imperfections in seconds.

Powder

Loose is best as it gives the most **natural finish** and is easy to apply. It is also worth keeping a pressed powder compact in your handbag for daytime touch-ups.

Eyebrow pencil

Choose one that is the same colour as your brows and use it to fill in or **define** where needed.

Eyeliner

Choose a **soft textured** pencil that can be applied easily and quickly.

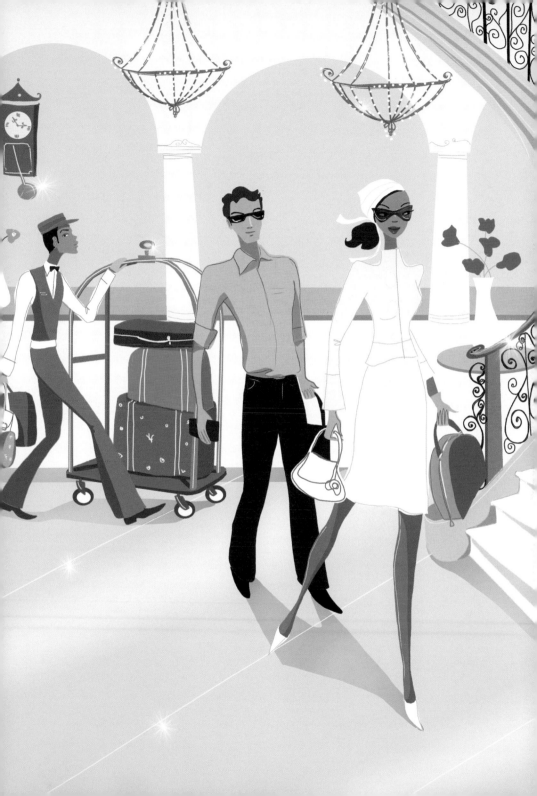

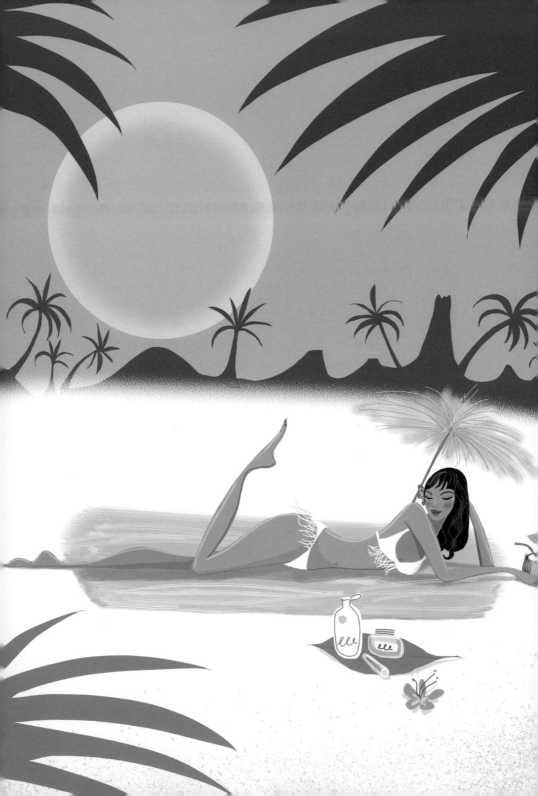

Eyeshadow

Have one **everyday colour** and one shimmery signature shade for evenings. Shading and blending are best left to make-up artists, so stick to one or two shade combinations to keep it simple.

Blusher

The right shade will make you look **younger** and **healthier**. Cream and gel blushes are the fastest and easiest to apply.

Lip pencil

Save this for **evenings** out, as applying it is too time-consuming for everyday make-up.

Lipstick

Forget fiddling around with brushes! Using lipstick **straight from the tube** is so much easier and just as effective. Make sure you have one neutral shade and one more daring and sexy evening colour.

Mascara

Wear this everyday for **eye definition** and longer lashes. Choose lengthening formulations that are also waterproof, so you don't need to worry about re-applying or under-eye smudging during the day.

Desert island glamour

If you were stranded in the middle of nowhere, what are the three products you couldn't live without? Learning what you can manage without will help teach you grooming shortcuts and make you a true beauty survivor.

DOUBLE-DUTY BEAUTY

When you're in a hurry, or have limited handbag space, two-in-one or **multi-use products** can be a lifesaver. Here are a few tricks to try.

✿ **Bronzing** powder and **Vaseline** can be used to make up a whole face with a bit of creativity. Use the bronzer dry as blusher and eyeshadow, then mix with a little Vaseline to create **lip gloss**. Finally, a slick of Vaseline on lashes and brows will complete the groomed look.

✿ Invest in some **three-in-one sticks**, which are meant to be used on lips, cheeks and eyes, for matching make-up in a flash.

✿ Brown mascara can be used on brows for grooming and **definition** as well as on lashes.

✿ Keep a packet of **three-in-one face wipes** that cleanse, tone and moisturize for those moments when you have neither the time nor the energy to use three products.

MAKE-UP COUNTDOWN

You've heard of painting by numbers? Follow these steps to putting on make-up in minutes. The less time you have, the more steps you can skip.

10 Cleanse
Use facial wipes for a speedy clean.

9 Moisturize
Apply a light moisturizer and blot after 2 minutes to remove excess.

8 Apply foundation
Tinted moisturizers are fast to blend and add instant colour.

7 Cover up
A cream version blends easily and can be used solo, without foundation.

6 Colour the cheeks
Apply colour to just the apples of the cheeks for a fresh-faced blush.

5 Focus on the eyes
Use a lighter colour on the browbone and a deeper tone in the crease.

4 Enhance lashes
Choose lengthening mascara for maximum impact.

3 Groom brows
Use a special brow comb to groom brows into shape.

2 Add lip colour
Sheer formulas and glosses are easiest to apply in a hurry.

1 Set and go
Finish off with a dusting of loose translucent powder.

QUICK DATE BEAUTY

He's ringing the doorbell but you're not anywhere near presentable, much less feeling confident, sexy and attractive. Luckily, there are ways to remedy this situation and turn it around quickly in your favour. Remain calm and regain the upper hand by remembering a few beauty basics. First, **look fresh** and **clean** – or at least give the impression that you are! And now comes the tricky part. You will need some **clever skills** to turn yourself into a **sexy siren** before his eyes and you will need to do it fast. Because he's here to spend time with you, not on his own while you're locked in the bathroom for hours.

Pay particular attention to your skin – with luck, more of it may get revealed later on! **Moisturize** any rough areas, as well as those on display, like the décolletage, legs, heels (especially if you are wearing sling-backs or strappy sandals) and hands. Next, quickly touch up your face. Apply a **radiance booster**, cover any dark circles or spots with concealer and then move onto the eyes, cheeks and lips. You will not have time for make-up brushes, so instead use a multipurpose stick (see page 270) before finishing with mascara. Unless your hair is dripping wet and really needs drying, simply brush and go.

Desperate measures

1 **Forget the shower, freshen up with a couple of baby wipes, a squirt of deodorant and scent.**
2 **Pull dirty hair off your face. This will make you look fresh-faced and clean, even if you don't feel it!**
3 **If your nail polish is chipped, simply remove it and go nude. Give your nails a quick scrub first, though.**
4 **If you don't have access to toothpaste, chew gum or crunch a couple of mints for instantly fresher breath.**

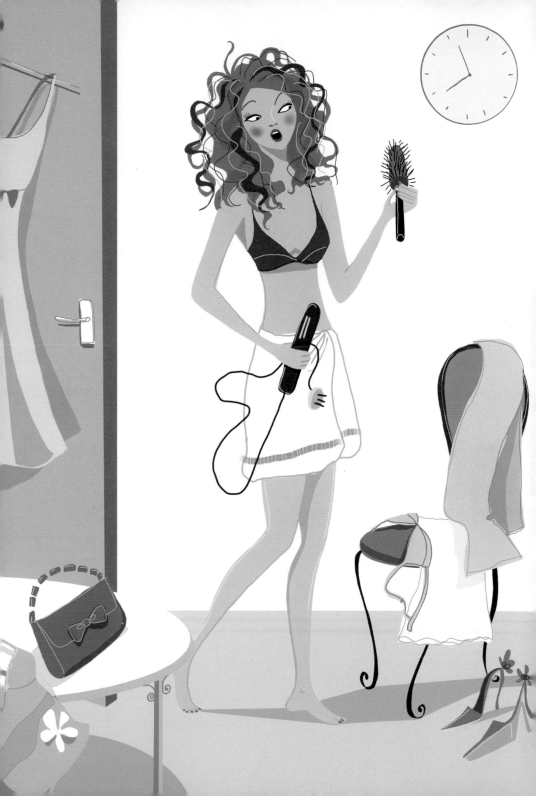

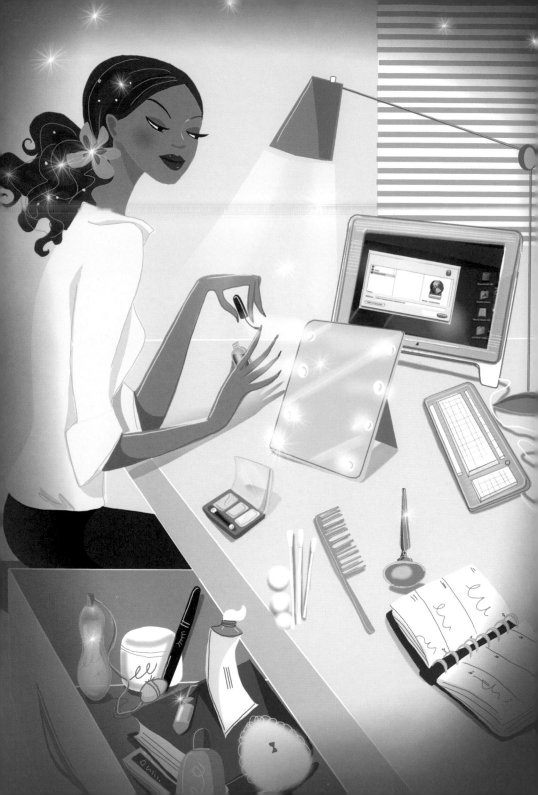

OFFICE TO PARTY BEAUTY

We've all spent ages queuing for the office toilets in order to get a bit of mirror space so we can apply make-up for a party or after-work do, only to end up slapping it on in a hurry. Read on to discover how you can **transform your look** in 10 minutes and avoid arriving flustered and unkempt.

HAIR

✿ Nothing beats an 'up-do' for **transforming** a daytime look into night, so make sure you wash your hair the morning of the party. Contrary to popular belief, freshly washed hair is easier to put up as it has a great deal more volume.

✿ For **speedy style**, working from the crown, simply take random sections of your hair, backcomb a little at the roots, twist and pin to your scalp using hair grips. You should only need eight sections for the whole head. This is a loose, modern look, so don't worry about making it perfect and leave the ends sticking out. The result should be sexy but stylish.

✿ To give your hair more hold, **spritz** each section with hairspray before pinning it. Choose a product that contains shine agents to leave hair ultra-glossy.

✿ For instant evening **glamour** put a few diamanté hair jewels in your hair. Dot them around so they catch the light and sparkle whenever you move your head.

MAKE-UP

✿ The three magic places to apply **bronzer** are the forehead, nose and chin. They are the areas that normally catch the sun, so a light dusting of bronzing powder, applied with a big brush, creates a natural looking, but instant glow.

✿ Don't worry if there isn't time to draw a perfect, wobble-free line with eyeliner, try this clever cheat instead: Draw several small dots along the top of your eyelid, close to the lashes, and then smudge them into a continuous line using a cotton bud (Q-Tip) or your finger. The result? **Smouldering party eyes**.

✿ For sexy lashes, fast, heated **eyelash curlers** are a must. They really open up the eyes and, when combined with the latest double-ended mascaras, create a dramatic effect. Put your mascara on first and it will act as a setting agent for the curlers so the effects last longer.

✿ Varnished nails make you look instantly more groomed, but can take hours to dry. Solve the problem by using one of the latest **fast-drying polishes** to paint your nails while sitting at your computer.

✿ And for last-minute grooming use a quick slick of **Vaseline**. It is so versatile and can be used just about anywhere – tidying eyebrows, glossing lips, and if you run some along your collarbone and calves, as it catches the light it creates the **illusion** of slimness.

★ TIP To prevent embarrassing 'lipstick on teeth' moments, put your thumb in your mouth after applying your lipstick and then pull it out slowly. This will remove any excess colour.

Maintenance Checks

Safeguard against 'bad everything' days by being a good-maintenance girl.

★ Set a regular evening each week to check out the state of your body, face and hair, then book any treatments accordingly – for example, check your legs, bikini area, and any other potentially overgrown spots that need waxing.

★ Once a week, check if any of your everyday products are running out and replace them straight away so they will be there when you need them.

★ Keep a basic make-up kit in your handbag as well as at home for fast fixes.

STREAMLINE YOUR BEAUTY BOX

We all hoard make-up – some of it years old – but having a good clear-out will **save you lots of time** searching for products in the morning. Doing this will also stop you getting stuck in a make-up rut, using the same lipsticks and eyeshadows everyday just because they're handy. Follow this three-stage plan to get things in shape.

BANISH BUGS

Most products have a **shelf life** of two years, with the exception of mascara, which should be replaced every three to six months to prevent eye infections. Throw out any foundations, moisturizers or nail polishes that have separated. If you're not sure how long you have had a product do the 'sniff test': if it doesn't smell right, it's probably past its sell-by date.

IF YOU DON'T USE IT, LOSE IT

Get rid of any products that you haven't used in the last year. A few items, such as glittery eyeshadow and bright red lippy, are fine to keep for special occasions, but **be ruthless** with everything else. Any lipstick – no matter how expensive – that you always end up wiping off because it just doesn't look right, needs to go.

GET BACK TO BASICS

Keep things simple. Identify the everyday **essentials** that you know suit you and stick to them, updating every now and again with well-chosen new products.

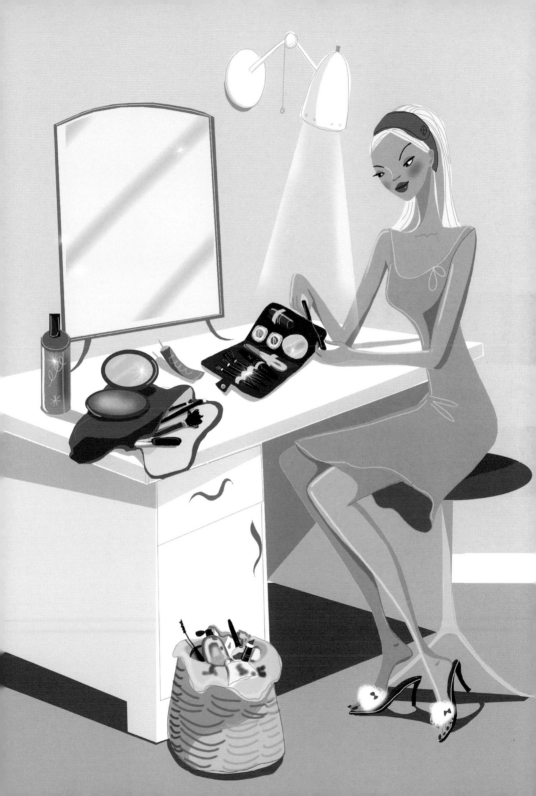

MAKE-UP SOS: HOW TO SOLVE THOSE LAST-MINUTE DISASTERS

TOO **DARK FOUNDATION**

If you have time, remove it and start again. Failing that, use a **face wipe** to lighten and blend in the foundation, paying special attention around the jaw and hairline to get rid of any tell-tale tidemarks.

FLAKY CONCEALER

If make-up is making a spot look dry and flaky, clean it off and hold a warm, damp cloth against it, rubbing gently. Remove any remaining flakes with tweezers, smooth the area with oil-free **moisturizer** and finally apply a little concealer with a clean lipstick brush, sealing with a tiny bit of powder.

TOO MUCH **BLUSHER**

Rub gently, in a circular motion, using a cotton wool ball dipped in loose powder. Then sweep a **clean powder brush** over the apples of your cheeks to further soften the colour intensity.

SPIDER-LEGS MASCARA

Don't apply more in the hope that it will even things out as it will only clog your lashes up more. Instead, wait until the mascara is dry, and then **comb through** with a lash comb until the excess is gone.

SMUDGED MASCARA

If it is not waterproof, a wet cotton bud (swab) will easily **wipe off the mistake**. For the waterproof variety, dip the cotton bud into eye make-up remover and gently rub it off.

WOBBLY LIQUID EYELINER

If you're in a hurry and don't have time to clean it off and reapply, turn it into the **smoky eye look**. Wait until it's dry and then blend it with a damp eyeshadow brush until it forms a soft, smudgy line.

STREAKY SELF-TAN

Jump straight into the **shower** and, with a **loofah** or a salt- or sugar-based body scrub, slough off as much fake tan as possible. Afterwards, if you need to, use a wash-off tinted body make-up to even out the colour and a tinted moisturizer to do the same on your face.

FIVE OCCASIONS WHEN YOU NEED A PERFECT FACE – FAST

THE SCENARIO
You want to look awake for the morning meeting at work

When you're short on time, getting your skin looking its best should always be your main priority. Spend a couple of minutes applying foundation and/or concealer to even out skin tone and hide blemishes and dark circles. Set everything with a flick of loose powder and, if you have time, apply a layer of mascara and a natural shade of lipstick.

THE SCENARIO
You want to look polished for a job interview

The key is not to look flustered – even if you have rushed like crazy to get there on time. Keep it simple so you can spent the time you do have perfecting the finer details, such as applying fast-dry nail polish and tidying your eyebrows to create a groomed, professional finish.

THE SCENARIO
You want to look glamorous for after-work drinks

No time to take off your daytime make-up and start all over again? Don't worry, simply refresh the skin with a facial spritz (a face toner in a spray bottle), reapply concealer to under-eye bags and spots, and tidy up under your eyes with a cotton bud (Q-Tip) dipped in eye make-up remover. Then intensify your existing make-up by adding another layer of colour to your cheeks and eyes and finish with plenty of lip gloss.

THE SCENARIO
You want to look SEXY for a romantic tête-à-tête

When you're trying to impress a new man, it's important to strike a balance between subtlety and glamour. You want to look good, but not like you tried too hard. Make sure that your skin is well moisturized and looks flawless – choose a light-reflecting foundation to create a flattering effect. Then concentrate on the eyes and combine smoky shadow colours with softly smudged eyeliner and lashings of mascara for a smouldering look. Keep lips and cheeks rosy but not too red, and avoid using too much lip gloss if you're planning to be kissed!

THE SCENARIO
You want to look fresh-faced girl-next-door for meeting the parents

The golden rule here is to keep your make-up natural-looking; the last thing his parents want to see is their son with an 'over-made-up hussy'. For a healthy glow, opt for tinted moisturizer rather than heavy foundation, and use a little concealer under the eyes so you don't look like you've been out partying all night, even if you have. A touch of cream blusher will add a rosy glow. Finish with one coat of mascara and some tinted lip gloss.

★ **TIP** Keep a cream concealer and lip brush in your make-up bag at all times to cover spots and eyebags if you're caught on the hop without any make-up.

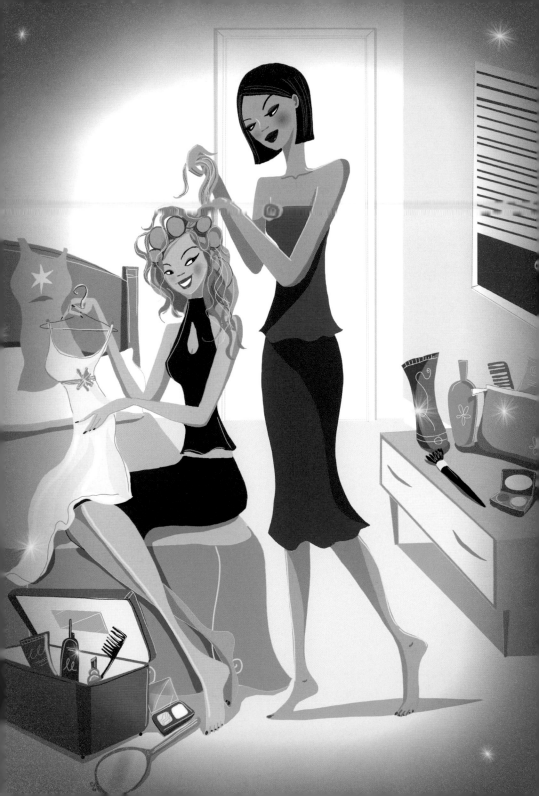

GET YOUR OWN **PERSONAL** ASSISTANT

For those special occasions you just can't face alone, whether it's a party where the ex will be with his new girlfriend or a black-tie fund-raiser with a high celeb count, beg your best friend to be your hair and make-up artist. She can advise on your look, help calm your nerves and make clear, objective choices at a point when your decision-making is yo-yoing and your stomach is fluttering. She will be sure to steer you in the right direction and won't let you go out looking foolish or fat. Here's a schedule to help you manage your time in the days and hours before the big event.

3 days ahead

Plan your outfit, make-up and hair. Make sure you've got all the supplies you need.

1 day before

Go for a manicure, pedicure, facial and skin-smoothing treatment or massage. This will make you feel relaxed, pampered and ready for anything.

3 hours before

Blow-dry your hair like the professionals: apply a little mousse or styling lotion, divide your hair into sections and dry it section by section. Finish with a spritz of high-shine serum for star-like gloss.

2 hours before

Apply body lotion, concentrating on problem areas such as knees and elbows. Use one that contains shimmery light-reflecting particles if your skin will be on show.

1 hour before

Star on the final stage – make-up. Begin with foundation, then eyes, lips and finally paint on the perfect pout, using a lip fixer for maximum staying power.

HOW TO BE A
BEAUTY REBEL

There are so many dos and don'ts, musts and shouldn'ts when it comes to looking good – following them all can be time-consuming, not to mention exhausting! But take heart, some **rules** were **meant to be broken** – here are the ones you can get away with ditching.

WEAR STRONG EYE MAKE-UP OR STRONG LIPSTICK, **NEVER BOTH** TOGETHER

There is no reason why you can't wear full-face make-up that doesn't look over-the-top. Simply choose **neutral colours** that let your natural skin tone show through. Sheer cream or gloss eyeshadows are good choices, as are lip glosses. Both add a wash of colour without looking too severe.

ALWAYS USE **POWDER OVER FOUNDATION**

The idea of using powder to 'set' your foundation is now considered very old-fashioned and can actually make you look much older than you are. Your base is meant to even out your skin tone, not to mask it, so **natural is best**. Use powder sparingly to blot a shiny T-zone.

ALWAYS **MATCH** YOUR **FINGER- AND TOENAILS**

Yet another outdated tradition. These days it's not cool to look like you're trying too hard, so instead of matching your fingers and toes choose **colours that coordinate**. In general, lighter colours look best on fingers for everyday while toenails suit deeper, richer shades.

USE LIP **PENCIL** TO CONTAIN YOUR **LIPSTICK**

A natural, sexy pout doesn't have a hard edge around it. Long-lasting lipsticks are so effective these days that it is not necessary to try and stop it smudging. **Pillar box red** lipstick is probably the only time when lip liner can still be of use as this colour will always be prone to bleeding into the fine lines around the mouth.

NEVER PUT **MOISTURIZER OVER** YOUR **MAKE-UP**

The newest oil-free moisturizers are so light they won't disturb your make-up or block your pores, so there is no harm in applying a little lotion here and there for **extra dewiness** during the day.

LET YOUR NAILS 'BREATHE' BY HAVING **POLISH-FREE** WEEKS

Nails are dead, so they can't breathe! Keeping them polished actually provides an extra layer of protection against **splitting and breakages**, but do give your nails the once over when you clean polish off to check for ridges or any white or green spots that could suggest a fungal infection. If they just look a bit yellowish it will simply be staining from the nail polish, so make sure you wear a base coat to prevent this.

WOMEN SHOULD **CUT THEIR HAIR** SHORT **ONCE THEY PASS 30**

With 30 being the new 20, who's to say what hairstyle anyone should have? The common belief is that longer styles can look heavy and drag the face down, thus ageing it. But if you choose a layered, **shaped style** with plenty of texture and keep your hair in good condition, there is nothing to say that you can't keep it long until you are 90!

YOUR **ROOTS** SHOULD **NEVER SHOW**

Darker roots or darker-coloured hair underneath can be a fashion statement. It **can add depth** and, done correctly, looks like the result of nature, not neglect – curly or layered hair carries off the two-tone effect best. What never looks good, however, is peroxide blonde hair with two inches of dark brown regrowth.

NEVER PULL OUT **GREY HAIRS**

It is a myth that pulling out one grey hair means it will be replaced by **ten new ones**. Tweezing the odd grey strand is harmless, but if you are talking about more than a few you're better off having a colour treatment to hide them rather than pulling them all out!

INSTANT **FACELIFT TRICKS**

Sadly, some ageing is inevitable, but there are things we can do to minimize the damage and cleverly **conceal the years**. Here is how to look ten years younger in as many minutes – no surgery required!

Apply a little cream pearl highlighter to your browbone, top of cheekbones, and in the inside corner of the eyes. This will make you look **younger** and more fresh-faced.

Brighten droopy eyes. Grooming eyebrows with careful waxing and plucking gives the **illusion of lifted lids** and having more skin showing at the browbone opens up the entire eye for a younger look.

Try skin-brightening face creams. These are designed to tighten your complexion and leave skin looking healthier and **more radiant**, knocking off years in the process.

Smile! Stop worrying about laughter lines. Because our faces lose fat as we age and our brows become lower, in repose we tend to look more serious, unhappy, or even cross. When you smile, your face lifts immediately and your cheeks, which may have hollowed, become instantly rounder and more youthful.

Go **easy on the mascara** and don't coat your bottom lashes – there's nothing more ageing than the spidery, clogged-lash effect.

SHORTCUTS TO YOUNGER SKIN, WHATEVER YOUR AGE

YOUR TWENTIES

Your skin should be more stable now than it was in your teens. Problems, such as oiliness and spots, will hopefully lessen, although adult acne is on the increase and has been linked to high stress levels. Your lips are plump, with no lines around them, and there are few, if any, wrinkles around your eyes. Your skin is functioning well but needs protection from the sun to prevent cell damage that will show up later in life. Good skincare habits should begin now.

What you can do

✿ Wear at least SPF25 every day.

✿ Use a separate eye cream to start protecting the delicate eye area.

✿ You can get away with most make-up but remember, your best look is probably a natural one using tinted moisturizer, eye and cheek creams, and lip gloss.

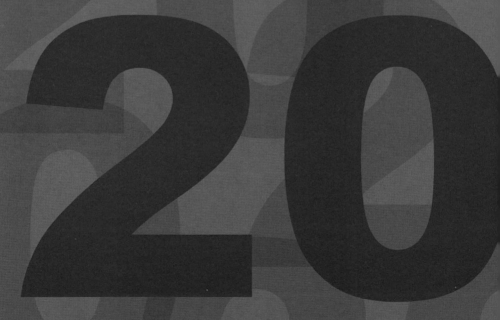

YOUR **THIRTIES**

Your thirties is the time when skin may start to lose some of its youthful bloom, as cell turnover slows. Smoke, alcohol, pollution and UV light all cause premature ageing and overexposure to any of them during your twenties will now begin to take its toll in the form of fine lines around the eyes and mouth. Collagen and elastin in the skin get weaker and wrinkles start to form as 'expression' lines. Skin looks generally duller than before and probably takes longer to recover from late nights or stress.

What you can do

✿ Use SPF25 daily and wear a hat or stay in the shade on holiday.

✿ Change to a richer moisturizer.

✿ To help brighten skin, slough off dead cells using a product containing alpha-hydroxy acid (AHAs).

✿ Don't wear heavy make-up. Choose cream-to-powder eyeshadows, cheek and lip stains, and matt lipsticks.

YOUR **FORTIES**

The rate at which your skin renews itself will really slow down in your forties. Any signs of tiredness will now show immediately in your face and thread veins may become more obvious. Your circulation and lymphatic drainage systems will slow too, which may cause puffiness around the eyes. Hormones play the biggest role around the time of the menopause and the drop in oestrogen levels can make skin thin and dry.

What you can do

✿ Use SPF25 to protect skin from the sun and prevent any further cell damage occurring.

✿ Treat yourself to monthly facials to keep your skin in good condition.

✿ Use a cream containing Retinol to exfoliate and reduce fine lines.

✿ Avoid dark lip and eye make-up as they accentuate lines. Go for peaches, pinks, and beiges instead and try a light-reflecting foundation.

YOUR **FIFTIES**

If you haven't protected your skin, sun damage will now be apparent in the form of wrinkles, spider veins and patches of pigmentation. You may notice an apparent increase in the size of your pores – they haven't got bigger, however, the skin around them has simply thickened, making them look more pronounced. Decreased oestrogen levels slow down sebum production and make the skin drier.

What you can do

- ✿ See a skin specialist to determine your skin's needs – they will be very different now.
- ✿ Apply a rich moisturizer containing SPF25, as continued protection from the sun will prevent any further damage.
- ✿ If you choose to relax wrinkles using Botox, make sure you see an experienced doctor as side effects can include droopy eyes.
- ✿ Your make-up should gently enhance your features. Go for a light-reflective base and pale lip colours. Avoid powder eyeshadows as they sit in the wrinkles around the eyes and accentuate them.

THE **FOUR MAGIC INGREDIENTS** FOR **YOUNGER-LOOKING** SKIN

Burning the candle at both ends, with work and a hectic social life, can mean your skin needs a little extra help. Look out for the following ingredients in your skincare range, as science has found that they can lend a helping hand in the fight against ageing. If you experience any soreness or skin irritation, discontinue using a product immediately.

VITAMIN A

It can help **diminish** the depth of wrinkles, thanks to its inflammatory action, which plumps up the skin to make wrinkles look less deep.

VITAMIN C

It has a **brightening** effect as it can help to boost circulation and increase the skin's production of collagen.

ALPHA-HYDROXY ACIDS
(AHAS OR 'FRUIT ACIDS')

They improve the skin's appearance by speeding up the shedding of old, dead cells from the skin surface, revealing the **fresher**, younger-looking skin underneath.

RETINOIDS

These are chemicals that encourage the skin produce new cells more quickly, making it thicker and more compact. After a month or two of use, the skin becomes **smoother** and fine wrinkles are reduced, but after six months this reaches a plateau and your skin won't continue improving. If you discontinue use, the skin reverts to its previous condition. Sadly, it will have no effect on deeper lines.

LOOKING AFTER HAIR IN A **HURRY**

Good care and styling tricks make for great-looking hair. Master these techniques and bad hair days will become a thing of the past – even when you're in a morning rush. Paying a bit more attention to your hair regime will save time in the long run.

SHAMPOO

Think you know how to shampoo your hair? Maybe you could do it better. To get the very best from your shampoo you need **even distribution**. Make sure you use the pads of your fingers, rather than your nails, to prevent scratching your scalp and, most importantly, never ever shampoo your hair in your bathwater. You should always use clean water for the final rinse. You can wash your hair every day, even twice a day, as long as you use a good-quality, mild shampoo.

APPLY **CONDITIONER**

The type of conditioner you use will depend on your hair type, but when it comes to application concentrate on the **mid-lengths to ends** only. Do not make the mistake of applying your conditioner as you would your shampoo. Use a comb to distribute it evenly throughout the hair and be sure to rinse it out thoroughly, as any residue will leave hair looking dull.

CREATING **TEXTURE**

Applying wax to damp hair locks in moisture and creates a shiny, glossy look. Use it on dry hair and you will achieve a textured finish. For the best results add just a small amount of wax at a time and **gradually build it up** until you get the desired effect. Remember it is much harder to remove than apply, so in this case less is more.

STYLING **SHORT** HAIR

Getting short hair to stand tall is easy when you know how. For fuss-free styling, fast dry hair with your fingers. Take sections of hair, hold vertically and spray with hairspray to fix. Go lightly at first and spray more if you need extra hold. You can also blow-dry the spray before it sets to fix the hair in place. This is especially good for fringes.

GETTING **ROOT LIFT**

If you want to add plenty of 'oomph' to your style you need to get right into the roots. Apply mousse to damp hair at the root area before you blow-dry. Try tipping your head forward so you can get straight to the area you want to lift.

ADDING **MOVEMENT**

Getting long hair to do anything but hang can be tricky. For lots of movement try spritzing hair with hair spray, then rake your fingers through as you blast dry. Finally, brush hair to ensure plenty of swing. Always use your hairdryer on the lowest and hottest settings, as this will help your hair to keep its natural body.

QUICK TIPS FOR
HEALTHY HAIR

✿ **Regular trims** are a must in order to keep hair in tip-top condition. Try to go every six to eight weeks and you should avoid that 'in-between' stage where hair goes straggly and loses its shape. Spending time in the salon will save you time and hassle in the long-run as your hair will be easier to style in the morning when you're rushing to get ready.

✿ For maximum efficiency, choose a '**wash and go**' style that doesn't need fancy drying techniques or special hair-styling tools. Long, layered looks are great, as they can be kept quite simple for daytime and then jazzed up for the evening using curlers or straighteners to change the look. If you love short hair, again go for a versatile style that can be kept simple for work and then made funkier with gels or wax when you want to make a bit more of a statement.

✿ Once a week, use a **deep moisturizing treatment** to replenish and protect your hair. All hair types will benefit from this, but dry or coloured hair should be treated more frequently.

✿ If you spend hours each morning straightening your hair, think about **thermal reconditioning**, a treatment that works in the opposite way to a perm, by permanently flattening and smoothing the hair. Unlike the more old-fashioned 'relaxing' hair treatments, it uses heat – not just chemicals – to get the hair even straighter, plus it adds moisture to boost shine.

✿ Ask your hairdresser to give you a **blow-drying lesson** – many salons offer them now. He or she can teach you some of the tricks of the trade, so you can create salon-looking hair without leaving your house.

STYLE MANAGEMENT

Making decisions about your hair can require weeks of deliberation and countless discussions with your friends. Actually doing something about your hair requires even more **effort**. As a busy girl, you simply don't have time to get it wrong. Here's some quick ways to manage three hairstyling troublespots.

ASK FOR AN **EXTENSION**

Hair extensions have become so popular with celebrities in recent years that most salons now offer them. Though not a quick procedure, extensions are the ideal way to see what you'd look like with long hair and they can also help hair look better when it's in that difficult 'in between' growing-out stage.

PRACTISE THE PERFECT **'UP-DO'**

When your hair is dirty or just misbehaving, putting it up is a fail-safe option. The biggest mistake people make is that they try to do it all at once. The secret is to split hair into sections and use more than one clip. Preparing the hair first with a smoothing serum makes it easier to shape and means it won't go frizzy once it is up and in place. To make a bun or ponytail look modern, keep it loose and don't worry about any stray tendrils hanging down. Simply run a little wax over them so they look finished and not flyaway.

JOIN THE **BLONDE EXPRESS**

Express highlights: this clever idea involves having **two colourists** working together on your hair, applying highlights at the same time. As a result, arrival to leaving with your new colour takes approximately **half the time** it normally would. Many salons also offer 'express' treatments for facials, massages, and manicures and pedicures. Ask if you can combine your hair treatment with a body one for a super-quick makeover.

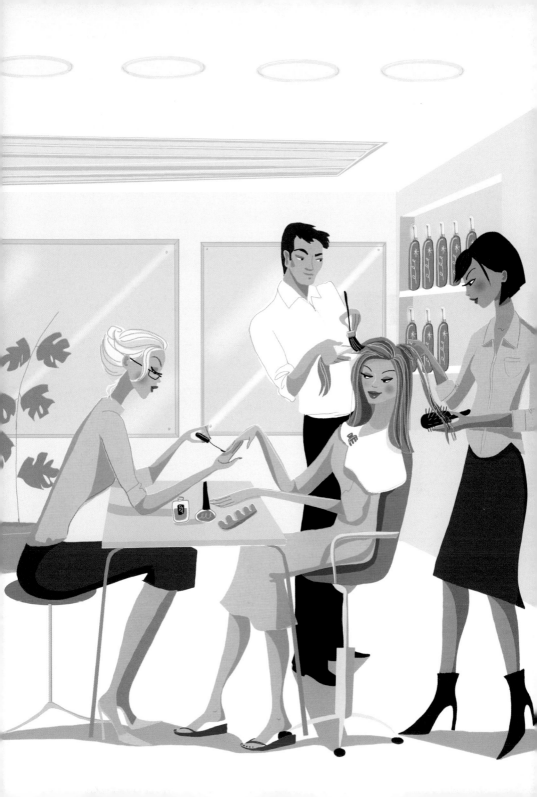

FAST WAYS TO TRANSFORM
BAD HAIR DAYS

When you go out in the morning knowing that your hair looks good
you feel confident and sure about yourself, but a 'bad hair day' can get
you off to the worst possible start ever. Here are a **few tricks** to help
you make sure your hair never lets you down.

PROBLEMS AND SOLUTIONS
Problem
Frizzy hair.

Solution
Don't brush it. Instead, rub a small blob of **smoothing
serum** between your palms and work it through your hair,
section by section. If your hair is curly use your fingers
to twist small pieces of hair into tight ringlets, then give
each ringlet a little tug so it hangs in a loose curl. If you
are blow-drying, wait 15 minutes before using a diffuser
to dry the curls; this will heat hair without lifting and
roughing up the cuticle.

Problem
Flat hair.

Solution
If your hair is looking flat and lifeless when you wake up, spritz it with water
to dampen it slightly, then **bend upside down** and, with your hands, scrunch
up handfuls of hair at the roots. Flick your head back up and you will have
instant lift and volume. If you have short hair, apply some **mousse to the
roots**, rub through and blast with your hairdryer on its hottest setting for
a few seconds. Leave it to cool before smoothing it back into shape.

Problem

Greasy hair.

Solution

If you don't have time to wash it try a dry **powder shampoo**. Sprinkle it liberally over the hair, concentrating on the roots, and work it through with your fingers. Leave it for a few minutes then brush it out. Dry shampoos contain a form of talc, which absorbs excess grease and makes hair easier to manage. If your hair still looks like an oil slick, tie it back or, if you have short locks, comb them away from your face with gel.

Problem

Dull hair.

Solution

If you have no time to wash your hair, spray a fine mist of **shine spray**, avoiding the root area, for instant gloss. If you have more time, wash your hair with a clarifying shampoo – it is designed to remove product and oil build-up. Blow-dry using a slanted nozzle and holding the dryer so that the hot air travels down and along the hair shaft rather than directly at it. This will help smooth the cuticles down, creating more shine in the process. It may also be worth investing in an **ionizing hairdryer** that claims to retain more of hair's natural moisture and thereby boost shine.

QUICK COLOUR TREATMENTS TO RETOUCH ROOTS

✿ If you have dark hair, ask your colourist if they can mix up a take-home **temporary colour** that you can use as a stopgap between visits.

✿ If you are going out but are worried about roots and don't have time to get your hair recoloured, pop to your nearest salon for **quick vegetable rinse** and blow-dry. This will add shine and help to disguise regrowth for a night out.

✿ If you haven't got enough time for a full or even a half head of highlights, ask your colourist for a '**t-section**' instead. This comprises of putting a few highlights around the side of your face and top of your crown and it only takes just over an hour – about half the time of a normal colouring session.

✿ If you have a grey hair emergency, applying a bit of **mascara**, in a matching shade to your hair colour, works as a handy SOS cover-up.

★ **TIP** If all else fails, a hat or headscarf will hide your roots, and you'll look chic and stylish.

Salon secret

Always wear gloves if you are colouring your hair
at home to prevent tell-tale stains on your hands.
If your home hair dye has stained the skin around
your face, dip cotton wool in baby oil, lemon juice,
or perfume and rub the mark gently. It should soon
disappear. In future, smooth a layer of Vaseline all
around your hairline before you start to prevent any
colour coming into contact with your skin.

THE **FIVE SECRETS** OF
MAINTAINING **COLOURED HAIR**

Follow these tips and your hair colour will stay **brighter** for longer, so you can save time and money by paying fewer visits to the hairdresser.

The more you wash your hair, the more your colour will fade. If you are used to **lathering up** on a daily basis and don't like to leave too long between washes, try alternating a shampoo day with a day of simply rinsing your hair with warm water.

Always use **conditioner**, even if you didn't need to before your hair was coloured. **Colouring damages hair**, leaving it porous and in need of more moisture to keep it looking healthy and shiny. Apply from just below the roots and massage through the hair lengths, concentrating on the ends. Always rinse off thoroughly.

Don't use styling mousse, gel or hairspray too often as they all contain colour-stripping alcohol.

Shun the sun. Sunlight breaks down hair colour, causing it to fade. To prevent this, **wear a headscarf** or hat on the beach and when walking around in sunny weather or apply a protective product that contains UV filters.

If your colour is looking a bit pale and jaded, extend its life with a **colour-enhancing shampoo** that will help to brighten it up.

Book ahead to avoid disappointment

Book in for your recolour while you are paying for your current hair appointment. This way you won't forget how long it's been and end up ringing for an appointment once your roots are already showing through. Make sure you write it in your diary straight away. It's amazing how many hair appointments get forgotten!

SPEEDY MANICURES

THE 5-MINUTE MANICURE

It is lovely having your nails done for you at the salon, but if you are short on time or money, home manicures are the answer. Make your manicure look as good as a professional one by following these three simple steps to the perfect polish:

PREPARATION

To begin with, take off any old colour with a good nail polish remover – acetone-free is the most gentle on your nails. Next, soak your nails in a bowl of warm water that contains a capful of liquid cuticle remover. Soak them for 3 minutes and, with a thin, dry flannel wrapped around your thumb, use it to push the cuticles back from your nails.

FILE AND BUFF

To shape your nails, choose a nonabrasive nail file – one that doesn't feel too rough to the touch. File the sides of the nail straight down and across the top. File in one direction only; never use a sawing, backwards and forwards motion as this will weaken your nails and make them more prone to splitting. Don't taper the nails into a point as this also makes them liable to breakages. Manicurists say the best shape for your nail is one that mirrors the shape of your cuticles. So, if your cuticles are rounded, your nail tips should be too. Next, buff nails with a three-way buffer. Buffing smooths the nail surface, stimulates nail growth and helps shift any leftover polish stains. Start with the roughest side, followed by the medium and finish with the smoothest to polish nails to a glass-like finish.

POLISH

Apply cuticle oil and massage in some hand cream, then run a nail varnish remover-soaked cotton pad over the nails to take off the greasy film, as this will prevent the polish adhering. First, apply a base coat, then apply two thin coats of your chosen colour, giving each layer a couple of minutes to dry in between. Finally, brush on a glossy topcoat to protect the nails and add shine. To make your manicure last, apply a layer of fast-drying topcoat every day.

TIME-SAVING NAIL CARE PRODUCTS

Mini nail file sticks can be kept in the tiniest of purses for emergency repairs.

60-second dry nail polish for glamorous nails without the wait.

Fast-dry topcoat or spray, so you don't have to sit still for hours in fear of nail smudges.

A pot of pre-soaked remover pads for removing chipped varnish on the train, bus or at your office desk.

A corrector pen to tackle last-minute mistakes before you leave home.

Tips for nail splits

★ Carry a file and clear nail polish at all times and keep nail glue handy to fix those 'below the quick' splits until they have a chance grow out.

★ If a nail does split very low down and a DIY job won't suffice, make an appointment at your nearest nail bar. They will be able to apply a silk wrap or acrylic tip over the nail and save it having to be trimmed.

FAKING IT:
HOW TO GET THE PERFECT TAN

What could be more time efficient than getting a golden tan in 10 minutes? Fake tanning products have become more and more popular as new research reveals just how much damage the real sun can do to our skins. Gone are the days of smelly, orange looking products that are hard to apply. Follow our foolproof plan to ensure a flawless finish every time.

SCRUB YOUR SKIN

Exfoliating is the most important process in preparing your skin to absorb fake tan. The more carefully you exfoliate, the better your tan will look as it is vital to remove all of the dead skin cells in order to prevent the tanning lotion from sticking to them and creating unsightly blotches.

Start by pampering yourself with a long soak in a nice warm bath to ensure that your skin is at its softest – a hot shower will do if you are in a hurry. Then, use an all-over body exfoliate, ensuring that all areas are scrubbed well in order to remove dead skin cells and unclog pores. It is essential that you pay particular attention to the knees, elbows and backs of the heels. These are the areas that are most prone to hard, dead skin and often give the fake tan game away. Using a body brush can also be very helpful for those hard-to-reach areas and will also help shift cellulite by increasing the blood circulation in affected areas. Make sure you exfoliate your face with a gentler product to prevent redness.

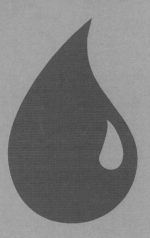

ADD SOME **MOISTURE**

You will now need to moisturize the entire area where you want the tan to appear. Some people claim that this isn't necessary, but others find it gives the most natural, even finish.

If you just want your face to be tanned then you only need to exfoliate and moisturize the face. If you require an all-over tan, however, then every single part of your body needs to be exfoliated and moisturized otherwise your skin will not absorb the tanning lotion. Start with your feet and work your way up to the face. Again, you will need to pay particular attention to the knees, elbows and heels – apply the moisturizer liberally. Use a different moisturizer for your face, as body creams tend to be heavier and can clog the facial pores.

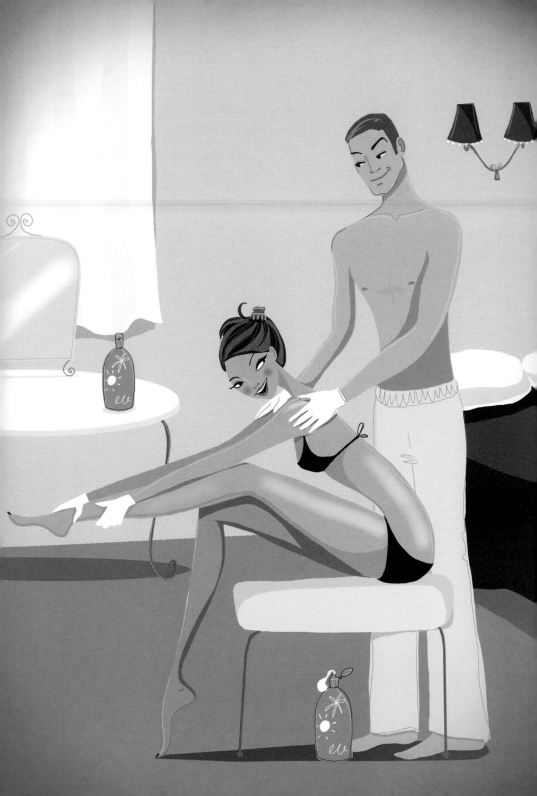

APPLY THE PRODUCT

It is best to apply fake tan with **protective gloves** to avoid streaky stains on your hands – the first tell-tale sign that your tan is not as genuine as you would like people to think! You can use surgical gloves, which often come with many self-tan products.

1 Starting with your legs, apply the fake tan according to the label's instructions. Rub the lotion into the skin with rapid movements. If you are not quick in your application at this stage the tanning lotion will absorb into your skin and leave you with unsightly streaking.

2 It is best to apply a very light application to your feet and hands, as these have awkward creases where the tanning solution can become uneven. Apply the lotion to the legs and use the 'film' of lotion that is left on your gloves afterwards to rub over your feet and ankles, ensuring that all movements are rapid so as to avoid any streaking.

3 At this stage, a cotton pad soaked in toner can be wiped over your knuckles, elbows and heels to prevent too much colour sinking.

4 Once you have blended the lotion into your legs and feet, you need to buff your skin, using your gloved hand, by very quickly going back and forth over the skin, buffing in any excess lotion to avoid patchy areas.

5 Repeat this process on your arms, but don't apply the lotion to your underarm or elbow; apply only to the top of the arm, making sure all the lotion is absorbed. Now rub the underarm and elbow with the remaining lotion left on the gloves, although no buffing is necessary here.

6 Finish the process by applying the lotion to your face, making sure that you do not apply too much and that the lotion is rubbed into the creases around the nose and just below the ears. Alternatively, you can use a product solely designed for use on the face.

★**TIP** You can apply a second coat of self-tan a couple of days later and from then on you should be able to apply the lotion once a week to maintain your golden tan. Exfoliate at least once a week to keep the colour even.

LUNCH-BREAK BEAUTY

Fitting in time for lengthy pampering treatments is not easy for most of us. Who hasn't sat in the hairdressers or at the nail bar looking at their watch and panicking about being late back to work or picking up the kids? Thankfully, most salons and spas offer express treatments for **busy women** who may have less than an hour at lunch in which to beautify themselves. Here are a few treats that may be on offer.

GREAT MAKE-UP

AT-THE-**COUNTER** MAKEOVERS

Many department stores and cosmetics boutiques offer makeovers. Although often free or redeemable against any products you buy, you will need to book if you're going over a lunchtime period. The staff are well acquainted with all the competing products on the market and can show you the latest colours and techniques – which will help you get out of a rut and away from all your 'safe bets'. Choose a brand that carries one of your favourite products, as you are more likely to be happy with their colours and textures.

GREAT SKIN

MICRODERMABRASION – A **MINI FACELIFT**
IN LESS THAN 60 MINUTES

This is a skin-polishing treatment designed to remove the top layer of dead skin in order to reveal the fresher, younger-looking skin beneath. It uses crushed microcrystals to gently lift off old cells, promote circulation, reduce the appearance of wrinkles and give skin an **instant boost**. It is also useful for spot-prone skin. The procedure is best avoided if you have sensitive skin, so check with your therapist.

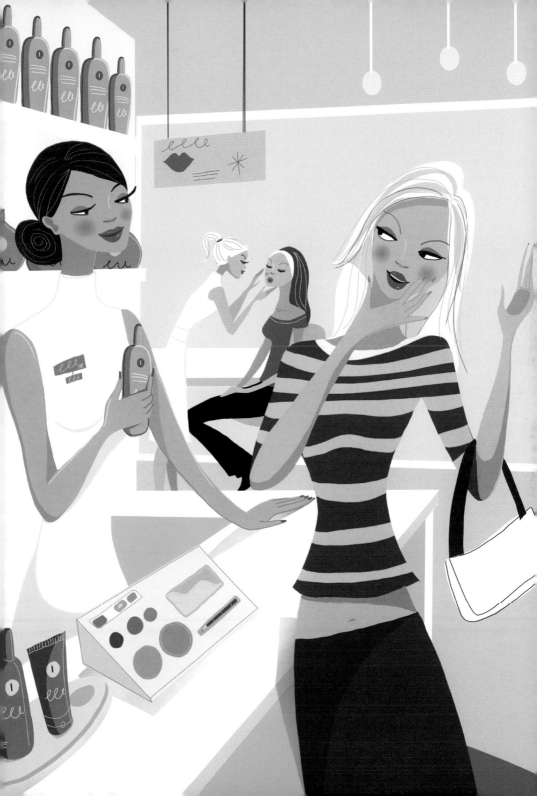

GREAT TAN

SPRAY TAN – LOOK **BRONZED** IN **3 MINUTES**

Many beauty salons are now offering spray-tan booths. You simply walk into them and then stand still while an **automatic jet of self-tan sprays** evenly over your whole body and face. The results last for up to a week and the shade and finish are both pretty natural.

GREAT TEETH

POWER-WHITENING – A **HOLLYWOOD SMILE** IN UNDER AN HOUR

If you drink coffee or smoke cigarettes, odds are your teeth could do with **brightening** up, even if you brush three times a day. The solution? Try a tooth-whitening treatment, which uses bleach to lighten the overall colour and remove stains – you can be in and out of the clinic in an hour, with your teeth an average of nine shades whiter.

GREAT HAIR

SPEED-DRY – 15 MINUTES TO **SLEEK, SMOOTH LOCKS**

A great idea if you're at work with dirty hair that needs restyling and receive an unexpected invitation to go out in the evening. Simply pop into your nearest salon and ask for a **super-fast wash and blow-dry** and you can be back at work, looking fabulous, in no time.

GREAT NAILS

THE 5-MINUTE MANICURE – A SWIFT ROUTE TO PERFECT NAILS

Manicures don't have to take 30 minutes. You'll find that most salons now offer a 'mini' version that involves a quick **reshape and polish**. If the salon has a selection of fast-dry polishes you could be out the door with great nails in around 5 minutes – which means that your boss won't even notice you've left your desk.

GREAT BODY

ALL-IN-ONE SALON PACKAGE

Book yourself in for a minibreak that offers a head-to-toe treatment in an hour, rather than the usual three-hour or day-long treatments. If you get one that includes a body massage, a facial and skin polish, you will be well on the way to glowing, smooth skin in no time, plus it's the perfect beautifying stress-reliever, especially if you go before a week in the sun or a big social event.

BEAUTY **TIME-SAVERS** OF THE **FUTURE**

New breakthroughs in the beauty world are **on the horizon**. Here are a few to look out for that are just around the corner.

THE **WRINKLE-FIGHTING** PATCH

In the past few years patches have become big business. We already have nicotine patches and patches for prescription drugs such as contraceptives that work by a process called a **transdermal delivery system** in which a paper-thin adhesive patch delivers time-released medication. Experts agree that it is a more **efficient** way to penetrate the skin than using a cream, which can wear off before the active ingredient has been **absorbed**. Researchers in the US are currently testing an anti-ageing patch to be worn on the face overnight, which contains line-busting ingredients such as vitamin C, collagen and green tea. So far, testers are reporting firmer, plumper skin after using them for just one night.

THE SHAMPOO THAT KNOCKS YEARS OFF YOUR HAIR

Hair companies are currently trying to develop a shampoo and conditioner that can bring back the **youthful bounciness** your hair had as a teenager. What's the point in feeding your skin with all the latest anti-ageing products only for your hair to reveal your true age? Once you hit your thirties your hair starts to lose its thickness and depth of colour, plus the follicles become weaker so more hair is shed and it doesn't always grow back. There are now plans to add the kind of ingredients, such as green tea and collagen, usually reserved for skin creams to hair products, in a bid for youthful locks.

THE END OF HAIR REMOVAL

Imagine never having to wax or shave your legs and bikini line ever again – how blissful! Although permanent hair removal is currently an option, it is only available in salons and it can cost a fortune. Scientists have now come up with a laser-type gadget that doesn't cost the earth and can be used in the **privacy** of your **own home**. The light-fuelled gadget works like a professional laser but is nowhere near as strong. It heats the hair follicles to slow their growth without any pain or skin damage, thus making shrieks and stubble a thing of the past.

THE **LIGHT** THAT **REVERSES AGEING**

Already available in some countries, treatment with light-emitting diodes (LEDs) – yes, the little lights that glow on your stereo – also known as '**photo modulation**', is one of the latest answers to holding back the clock. Research has found that the low-energy pulses of light given out by LEDs can improve skin tone, reverse sun damage and soften wrinkles. It appears to do this by stimulating the cells that produce collagen and elastin, vital elements in young-looking skin.

In contrast to other light treatments, such as laser, this new method doesn't heat or damage tissue, so there is no redness. One company called Techno-Lit is now working on creating a **home device** that utilizes this technology and hopes to make it available, and affordable, in the next few years.

THE NO-REDNESS
ACNE TREATMENT

Many topical creams make a great job of shifting
acne but, in the process, remove a layer of skin,
leaving your face red and sore. In the US, a new
topical antibiotic, Dapsone, has been found in trials
to quickly take the redness out of pimples. Testers
reported rapid **clearing of spots** with much less
irritation than with normal spot treatments.

THE INTELLIGENT
FOUNDATION

We now live in an age where
customized is cool, so the idea of
bespoke make-up, designed to
react to the individual wearer's
skin, is very appealing. Clinique is
currently developing a foundation
that uses '**mirror technology**',
in which tiny reflective particles
recognize and respond to lighter
or darker spots on your skin and
will cover or brighten them as
necessary. The result is a base that
looks perfectly sheer and covers
every imperfection.

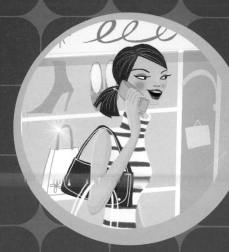

ACKNOWLEDGEMENTS

CAROLINE JONES THANKS:
Anita Pyre for her research skills.
I dedicate the book to my **mother** –
the **busiest girl** I know!

THE **PUBLISHERS** THANK:
Lucy Truman, and **Paula White**
at New Division.

USEFUL WEBSITES FOR
BUSY GIRLS

www.dailycandy.com
www.ediets.co
www.fitnessonline.com
www.health-fitness-tips.com
www.net-a-porter.com
www.sephora.com
www.spacenk.co.uk
www.weightlossresources.co.uk
www.weightwatchers.com

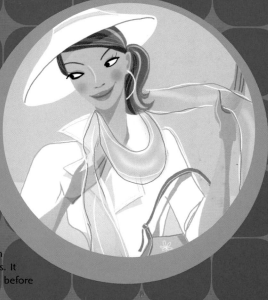

Publisher's Note
The information and opinions
contained within this book are
advisory only and may be of general
interest to the reader. This book is not
a substitute for professional advice on
nutrition, health, dieting or physical fitness. It
is advisable to consult with your doctor before
embarking on any diet or exercise regime.